NUTRITION MATTERS

PO Box 5253
1811 W. 2nd Street, Suite 435
Grand Island, NE 68802
(308)381-8361

Written Approval
requested and pending
from the following restaurants and franchises:

Amigo's	KFC
Arby's	Long John Silver's
Blimpie's	Max Magruder's
Boston Market	McDonald's
Burger King	Nonna's
Country Kitchen	Pizza Hut
Dairy Queen	Pump & Pantry
Denny's	Red Lobster
Driesbach's	Riverside Golf Club
Domino's	Runza
Farmer's Daughter	Sam's Club
Garden Cafe	Schlotzsky's Deli
Godfather's Pizza	Subway
Grand Island West Alda	Taco Bell
76 Restaurant	Taco Del Sol
Grandma Max's Restaurant	Taco John's
Habe'tat	Taylor's Steak House & Catering
Hardee's	U-Save Grocery Store
Hunan's	Village Inn
Imperial Palace	Wendy's
Incredible Bulk, The	Yen Ching
Interstate Holiday Inn	

**Reprinting any pages of
"How To Eat Healthy Wherever You Are"
by permission only.**

Special thanks to Omaha Methodist Hospital Dietary Department, for sharing A'fare of the Heart information for use in our book.

1

HOW TO EAT HEALTHY WHEREVER YOU ARE OR COUNT FOR YOUR HEALTH

In every revision of Count for Your Health, I try to include more current and practical information to help this small book be a major tool to identifying the issues of eating habits for each person who has begun to focus on their choices and healthy living.

There are two issues in beginning to change your eating style: knowledge of foods and available choices, and second record keeping of some type to give factual feedback and accountability. We need to be accountable till the changes become habits. These are not easy feats. The more consistent the records, the greater the chance to be honest about actual calories and fat averages being taken in.

Count for your Health is designed to help you first become aware of the calories and fat in your daily diet. Once you have learned what you actually eat, then you will be able to develop an individual food plan, with honest facts and NO guilt. Your goal weight, age, activity level and present health concerns need to be considered when deciding on a safe and effective range of calorie points and fat grams for YOU. Nutrition knowledge and your personal attitude are key factors in determining your success at weight control, and even more important your health.

Lowering calories and fat will mean shedding excess pounds, and lowering cholesterol. This flexible eating plan will reinforce your decisions to eat a variety of foods while you enjoy a lifetime of healthy eating. There is no diet to fall off of. Read the following information to set your calorie points and fat grams. The first two weeks you should record fat grams or calorie points! Doing both at the start may be too much, and too confusing.

Calorie Points and fat grams in this booklet are estimations only, from reliable and yet general information sources. If your portions are accurate, these estimations will be enough. YOUR ACTIONS AND ATTITUDE ARE EVERYTHING IN DETERMINING YOUR RESULTS!

KAREN BENSON RDCN
NUTRITION MATTERS INC 1996

WHAT'S NEW...

In 1996 labels and nutrition information are almost there for the taking. But first you need to understand the key terms, nutrient numbers and body needs, to make the label mean something. Almost all foods should have a nutrition label and an ingredient list. The new label, NUTRITION FACTS gives you standard serving sizes for the product, total fat grams, cholesterol, sodium, a breakdown of carbohydrates content, and even protein. The daily value is a guide for 2000 or 2500 calories. For FAT, SAT FAT, CHOLES-TEROL, SODIUM, AND SUGARS choose products low in daily value percentages. Personally, I steer people to staying with grams since percentages of actual intake take time and study to comprehend. You want to simplify healthy eating not complicate it. If you don't have time, stay with serving size and fat grams as the two mainstays to check. Key words on labels are improved (see below). Because the FDA has restricted the rules products with these terms are very low in fat. Yet you may eat many healthy and acceptable foods that fit your taste buds and your health need without meeting the FDA regulations.

KEY WORDS	MEANING
Fat Free	Less than .5 gram of fat/serving
Low Fat	3 grams of fat or less/ serving
Lean	Less than 10 grams of fat, 4 grams sat fat and 95mg of cholesterol/serving
Light	1/3 less cal., no more than 1/2 the fat, or 1/2 the sodium of the regular product
Cholesterol Free	Less than 2 mg of cholesterol and 2 gr. or less of sat. fat/serving

Last, but not least, keep telling the managers or owners of any food establishment what you need for food and nutrition information to stay "On TRACK". Customers' needs are the "bread and butter" of any food place and even more they want you back. Because your health matters more than anything....

Karen @ NUTRITION MATTERS
05/96

CHANGING YOUR THINKING, CHANGING YOUR YEARS....

You may be among the majority in the Mid-west who read about health, joke about diets and "exercise", and wonder why it has to be a concern... that is until one family member or friend, or you are confronted with a health situation. This situation, minor or major, requires more than positive thinking. It may be weeks or months to recover basic health or former life-style. We have enough new information to fortify your thinking in a manner that can keep you young and thinking in a way that you want to participate in taking care of your body. We do not have to leave it to genetic and aging "chance".

Some simple yet "fortifying" actions to influence the way you believe and think:

I) Be around people who exercise or eat healthy foods regularly....Note their attitude, their energy....What can you role model, what part of their life-style would you like for yourself, and what daily or weekly scheduling do they do that keeps them on track.

2) Read Current Health Information. Other people may turn you off by the corniness of taking care of the body and eating what's good for you. A Health magazine will give you case studies from people in real life and research. Maybe more important it will give you a perspective to reconsider your own actions. Post a few thoughts, or phrases on your frig, and your desk, to create your own connection with published information.

3) Do a simple exercise plan and food plan for one month. In that 30 days try to make no decisions about continuing. Just act as though you believe it. Journal comments, feelings, and actions whenever you can. At 30 days you will have some strong beliefs about where you want to go.

4) Complete a family "wellness" tree. Review with parents, siblings, cousins other family just what the generations before lived with as far as health problems, illnesses that took their life, or shortened it in some way. When you look at the details of death age, and the illness type, you will make some decisions what part of a healthy plan needs to be applied to you.

5) Add rather than subtract. Do not immediately take away food, rather add one food, safe food such as your favorite snack complemented with fruit, or a low fat snack may help satisfy cravings and be non-depriving.

6) Tell someone healthy changes you are experimenting with and make a lunch date in one week to keep yourself honest with your plan and open to others.

THE ATHLETE IN YOU

Eating for energy and stamina should be the goal of any athlete previous to any event when we want to be at our best!

Years ago ball players traditionally downed a pre-game meal of steak and trimmings - now most athletes have learned the changes pay off in food choices.

Your success will be held back if you exercise strenuously with a stomach and intestinal track filled with food or waste. Planning ahead is part of the game.

A meal high in carbohydrates, low in protein and fat will digest quickly with more available energy. High sugar foods may lead to hunger and low blood sugar. Carbohydrates are the ideal energy for the body. A pre-competition meal high in complex carbohydrates is easy to plan and to digest. Athletes should eat a carbohydrate rich diet everyday to enhance muscle glycogen storage. We are very individual in our tolerance to food types and when we eat pre-event. You may be able to eat a sweet or bread product just prior to your game. Real sustained energy will depend on foods and meals from the 24 hours preceding.

Here are some basic guidelines to improve your performance:
1/2 cup water per 15 minutes of exercise is minimum.
1-2 cups of water 2 hours prior and 2 hours post event will keep you hydrated.
Avoid new or unusual foods before actual competition.
A sweet such as a granola bar or a candy bar has been found to be helpful only in long endurance events.
A large meal should be consumed only if 3-4 hours are allowed before the exercise.
Eat well the two meals previous to the event.
Some high carbohydrate snacks are:

2 slices of bread	1 bagel
1 cup pasta	A lean meat sandwich
1 medium sized baked potato	A low fat pasta salad
3 cups air-popped popcorn	Baked potato with broccoli and cheese
1 medium-sized apple	Chili or chicken noodle soup
1 medium-sized orange	Fruit or vegetable salad with crackers
1 cup vegetable juice	Lean casserole or stew

Healthy eating cannot assure you of winning the game, yet poor nutrition can limit your energy and your ability.

CORNERING THE CARB CRAZE...

Athletes depend on them, dieting women avoid them, and if you're typical you are not even sure what foods contain that nutrient called carbohydrate. Take this three question quiz and then keep reading. It may change how you eat, how you "DIET", and how you think of balanced yet light eating for you and your family.

Four Groups of Foods that contain carbohydrates are:

Examples of Refined carbohydrates are (3):

Reasons to increase carbohydrate in my daily eating plan are (3 or more):

Carbohydrates are basic healthy foods that come from plant sources. Vegetables and legumes, fruits, breads and grains are all practical yet high nutrient carbohydrate sources that athletes and people who care about weight, energy, and overall heart health depend on. The other "unknown" yet great source of carbs is milk - because the cow's diet is from plants or should we say "grass"! Once the grain is refined to white flour or the sugar beet to a granule we have a product that may not be bad, yet has lost some nutrients in most cases, and is absorbed much quicker. Corn syrup is the refined carbohydrate of the nineties, often labeled as a dextrose. These facts may spur your interest in increasing carbohydrates in your meals and snacks.

Complex carbohydrates contain fiber that stabilizes your blood sugar, gives you a full feeling, and decreases some cancer risk and total blood cholesterol.

Four to six fruits and vegetables per day with any combination of the two groups is a great challenge to master for starting to improve the food choices, and to lose weight and body fat.

Carbohydrates are not high calorie - at four calories/gram they have the same calories as a gram of protein, and less than half the calories of a gram of fat which has nine. Our moms attempts to decrease breads and potatoes were unnecessary when it came to weight control, necessary only for limiting the butter and gravy or fat we still love to add.

If athletes give 70% of their day's calories to carbohydrate sources, then we can work toward the same non-diet plan with a goal of 50%. Record a day of what you eat and highlight the carbohydrates. The healthier the intake, the more colorful the page!

THE ALMIGHTY SCALE AND LOSING WEIGHT!

Losing Weight is a second occupation for too many Americans today. We spend billions trying new schemes, pills and powders. To actually lose body fat and a healthy weight loss takes four ingredients: proper levels of calories and fat, increased activity and exercise, an attitude that this project is a priority for health reasons, and a personalized system. The following facts may be beneficial to setting up your own plan:

Seventy percent of those who lose and keep the extra pounds off have a exercise and eating plan.

Ninety five percent of dieters regain their weight.

Making a written plan, with weekly challenges and behavior and weight goals is essential. Show your initial scheme to a friend and refine, evaluate, just "WRITE" about you goals and actions as frequently as possible, yet weekly at a minimum. Planner pads or calendars are handy tools that keep you focused.

One to two pounds of weight loss per week is possible as an average loss over several weeks. It takes 3500 calorie deficit to lose one pound or 200 calories we did without or expended for seventeen days. A faster loss signifies more muscle and water loss which of course returns.

Five to ten percent weight loss or total weight is reasonable and healthy over 6 months. For example if you weigh 180 pounds, your goal may be to lose 9-18 pounds and maintain that loss and new life-style in the next 3 - 6 months.

If you have made caloric changes and yet aren't seeing results check your activity and exercise plan to see what you can increase. Going under 1200 calories for a female in general, and males below 1800 is not helpful in real fat loss. Double check your portions of favorite foods and common daily foods like cereal, the amount of margarine on toast, etc.

You'll want to read "CORNERING THE CARB CRAZE" to look at your carbohydrate understanding and "HEART HEALTH" for checking out dietary fat's role in all of this. Best of all a healthy weight loss plan will not leave you deprived and grouchy, rather with new choices and a few replacements to those old favorites you still have on occasion.

The benefits - More than we can mention....even 10% of excess weight loss can lower blood sugars, blood lipids, hypertension, while improving mobility, breathing, and self esteem. You deserve to maintain a body that not only works, but feels good.

THE RECIPE FOR A HEALTHY CHILD

The number of children who are overweight has almost doubled in the last 25 years. However, the number of calories children between 5 and 16 need (with their smaller bodies and higher nutrients needs) range between approximately 2,000 to 2,500 calories per day. Too many children do not engage in enough physical activity to counter-balance their food intake.

Technology has made America a more sedentary society. While kids of yesterday preferred outdoor play after school, such as a game of soccer or softball, kids today are more likely to stay indoors and watch television or play video games. Also, kids do not know how to balance their food choices. We need to teach kids the benefits of healthy eating.

To help reverse the trend toward obesity in children, consider these choices for the kids you work with.

* Motivate kids to get out and be active! Physical activity such as roller-blading, soccer, gymnastics or biking stimulates the use of muscles and promotes growth.

* Keep in mind that kids who are active in sports, for example, expend more energy than kids who are less active, and prepare food accordingly.

* Encourage kids to obtain 10 to 15 percent of their daily calories from protein rich foods, such as lean meat, poultry, and dairy products, which help growing bodies build and repair muscles and other tissues. In addition, kids' dietary intake should consist of plenty of foods high in micronutrients, such as B-vitamins, vitamin E, calcium, iron, and magnesium, which help form the body skeleton and control body processes.

* Don't be afraid to give kids sideline snacks during practice or games. Snack foods like crackers, juice, candy and ice cream help kids maintain an adequate supply of energy (or fuel) throughout the day. These snack foods contain simple or complex carbohydrates, which are broken down into glucose to provide kids' bodies with immediate fuel, or are stored as glycogen in their muscles to be used as needed to power them during physical activity.

* Remember that it's OK to eat any food if it's consumed in moderation, choosing and eating a wide variety of foods with different tastes and textures will help achieve a healthful, nutritious diet.

Encouraging children to balance their food choices and to engage in regular physical activity can help kids overcome the challenge of obesity and grow into healthy, active adults. In addition, teaching children the benefits of healthy eating while they are young will encourage healthy eating habits later in life.

YOU CAN MAKE THE SWITCH

... If you are ready to go to this "healthier" lifestyle that's promoted everywhere - then you must apply some daily food preparation techniques to see any change. In exercise it is easier to believe maybe - yet it should make sense to all of us that moving, working and toning the physical body is the only way of keeping the parts of our moving body that are energetic - energetic...

In food preparation you do not have to give up all your favorite foods, and really shouldn't. It will make this a "DIET" if you give up your foodstyle, and not a good diet at that.

Here are some substitution ideas that we find work:

You can decrease 1/3 of the fat or sugar in most baking, and some cooked recipes without major changes in the product. You will need to add moisture in the form of fat free sour cream, yogurt, fat free or light cream cheese, applesauce, fruit, or juices to keep the product moist.

When decreasing the sugar or fat, gradually increase the amount of the ingredient you are cutting, to give the tastebuds some time to adjust, and to experiment with seasonings and other flavors that will keep this a good product...

Cakes, fruit crisps, and similar baked products will take little experimentation, while the cookies seem very sensitive to any recipe changes.

Measuring is everything. If you and I cut 100+ calories in a food daily, in a year that can be 12# difference. Favorite foods and meats are among the foods we have on a daily basis that need factual measuring. You'll be surprised what a cup is!

There are many lower fat, lower sugar ingredients now that taste good... You'll need to try several fat free chips, or light margarine's to know which one is acceptable to you.

Replacing foods that you normally have and "crave" is important to prevent "deprived" feelings that after time lead to over eating. Sugar and fat are learned tastes, and eventually even you might prefer the lighter item.

TIPS TO GAINING CONTROL OF YOUR FOOD INTAKE

The following suggestions may help to "see the benefits" of lowering fat intake, without a rigid DIET.

1. Keep a food record daily for at least 1 month. Evaluate results weekly and try to learn from your high and low fat days.

2. Find a friend, co-worker, or family members to be accountable to. Even better challenge the support person(s) to begin their own course of healthier eating. The goal is to see who stays on the weekly plan, not who loses the most weight. **Weight loss is a symptom of healthy eating.**

3. Ask questions, check ingredients, read labels, and measure portions. Your hard work will pay off. **BE HONEST WITH YOURSELF ON PORTION CONTENT OF FOOD. AT HOME AND AT RESTAURANTS BIGGER HAS BECOME BETTER. THE GRADUAL INCREASE IN PORTION SIZE HAS COME UNNOTICED BY MOST, WHICH MANY TIMES CREATES EXCESS CALORIES, FAT, AND WEIGHT!**

4. Find out what you are doing right and work at more "healthy" food behaviors.

5. Get professional help if you're feeling defeated. **All of us need coaching from time to time. The extra support and factual information could be enough to give you lifelong results.**

6. **Plan, Plan, Plan,** and stay in the present. Set goal rewards, and be patient. Weight loss and lowering cholesterol is a time consuming project possible for all who believe they can make a difference in their health and self image.

EXERCISE , EATING AND EQUAL PARTS....

The data continues to come in that weight loss to be achieved permanently, for heart health and energy is always accompanied by a change in EXERCISE.....!!

In I994 Americans learned that exercise can be broken up through the day for ease, for schedules, and even for attitudes that can only discipline themselves for a few minutes in one time period. Not only did we learn there are benefits from even I0 minutes of activity- yet also that gardening, mowing the lawn, and other "home" work, counts as well.

People today are not always over eating, and yet may weigh more, and have more body fat and health risks than the generations before us, that took in more calories.

The reason is clear...their work and activity level was higher activity due to limited technology. My dishwasher is priceless to my life-style, yet every task even in our kitchen, our jobs, and our housework, that has been simplified by appliances and state of the art mechanics allows our bodies to rest even more.

So the choice is yours. Your health risks at any weight, are greater with a sit-still life-style. As a friend of mine in exercise physiology says, " a body in motion stays in motion." I would not want to imagine the life-style of many energetic friends of mine without activity. The time with our children, the moments of fresh air and sunshine, the fun of sports together, and the opposite vision of walls and being tied to a couch or chair is important. Visualize your activity and your exercise time each week and make sure it sounds realistic and enjoyable. You will lose body fat, inches and gain toning and muscle with consistent activity coordinated with your changes in fat and calories. This may begin to happen long before the "almighty scale" pointer even budges....

Balancing the food plan and activity in your life equals things out-no extreme diets, yet non compulsive exercise, a plan you can live with...wherever you are.....

HOW TO USE FAT GRAMS

The American Heart Association and other reliable medical associations agree that taking in 25-30% of your total daily calories from fat is sufficient for health, and yet low enough to see positive wellness changes. This level is appropriate for weight or fat loss, and to lower serum cholesterol levels. If you choose to go to a lower percentage of fat in your diet, you need the advice of a physician. Monitoring from a registered dietitian will assure adequate nutrition and satiety. Persons going to extremes in lowering their fat intake often end up overeating/or bingeing because of chronic hunger.

FAT GRAM GUIDELINE:

CALORIE LEVEL	25%	30%
1200	33	40
1300	36	43
1400	39	47
1500	42	50
1600	44	53
1700	47	57
1800	50	60
1900	53	63
2000	56	67
2100	58	70
2200	61	73

Important clues to staying with fat grams:

Give yourself time to get to a lower level of fat in the diet. Easily we can take in 200 grams of fat/day. A reasonable starting goal for a woman would be for a woman to achieve an average of 40 fat grams/day, or for men an average of 65 grams/day. This will take some time; find out your usual intake first and then set a moderate and reasonable goal to lower fat slowly.

Fat grams are a successful tool in weight loss when the individual allows adequate calories. A level of 12-1500 calories is the minimum recommended for most women, and 1800-2000 for most men. Again, remember to contact a dietitian or your physician for guidance at any calorie level below this, or if weight loss is averaging more than one to two pounds per week.

IN 1996 WE LISTED CALORIES AS WELL AS CALORIE POINTS. THE POINTS CONTINUE TO BE A GREAT METHOD, YET THOSE WHO WANT TO ADD SPECIFIC NUMBERS NOW HAVE THEM AVAILABLE. IT IS WISE TO CHECK CALORIE TOTALS OR CALORIE POINT TOTALS ONCE OR TWICE WEEKLY IF YOUR A "FAT GRAM EXPERT", IF YOU'RE NOT SEEING CHANGES YOU FELT WERE DESERVED AND TIMELY, AND IF YOU LIKE CONCENTRATED SWEETS AND FOODS CONTAINING LITTLE OR NO FAT!!!

HOW TO USE CALORIE POINTS

ONE CALORIE POINT = 75 CALORIES. MANY COMMON FOODS EQUAL ONE POINT. (i.e. one slice of bread, a medium size apple, an ounce of meat, an egg). Your daily goal with calorie points is to stay within a pre-set range, allowing a safe level of calories for physical and mental health, and yet flexibility in food choices.

CALORIE LEVEL AND POINTS

1200	16
1300	17.3
1400	18.6
1500	20
1600	21.3
1700	22.6
1800	24
1900	25.3
2000	26.6
2100	28
2200	29.3
2300	30.6
2400	32
2500	33.3
2600	34.6
2700	36

To figure the calorie points on an unlisted food item: just find out the calories per serving and use this equation:

Calories per serving divided by 75 = total points

For example 110 divided by 75 = 1.5 points

TABLE OF CONTENTS

PAGE

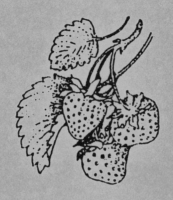

APPETIZERS

Careful is the Clue for these impulse, while you wait foods. . . .
Appetizers in restaurants are often fried and high fat, even those containing vegetables. . . .At home or for potlucks, you can make great choices and have something to take the edge off of a hearty appetite as a filler, and to satisfy chewing and the desire to have food in your hands when everyone else is eating.

Make a plan upon arrival of some limits on snack eating. Before you arrive is even better - for example:

1) Tonight nothing fried
2) I will stay within 10 fat grams for the party
3) I will eat fruit or a diet drink in between any other choices
4) I will get a small plate for appetizers at 8 and at 9, beyond this I will have to plan a healthy snack when I get home

Karen's Klue: My letter association for the work **PLAN**: any **P**rogress I make is **L**ed by my **A**ctions **N**ow!

My goal for you. . . .**NO REGRETS, REAL RESULTS.**

APPETIZERS

FOOD	AMOUNT	FAT GRAMS	CALORIE PTS	CALORIES
Anchovies	9 Fillets	3.5	1	75
Bacon	3 strips 2T.	7.2	1	75
Bked Bugle	42	2	1.2	90
Caviar	1 T	2	1	75
Cheetos, lt	34	6	1.5	112.5
Combos	1.8	10	2	150
Corn Nuts	1 oz.	4	1.8	135
DooDads	1/2 cup	6	2	150
Eagle Snack:				
Cheese cr	1 oz.	6	2	150
Pretzels	1 oz.	2	1.5	112.5
Egg Rolls	4 sm	6.8	2.5	187.5
Funyuns	1 oz.	6	2	150
Granola Bars:				
Archway	1 cookie	0	0.8	60
Betty Croc	1 pkg	8	2.25	169
Flavorkist	1	3	1.75	131
Kellogg's, L. Fat	1	2	1	75
Kudo Snack	1	12	2.66	199.5
N. Valley Bar	1	5	1.66	124.5
N. Valley L. Fat	1	2	1.5	112.5
Nutra Grain	1	5	2	150
Quaker Chewy, L. Fat	1	2	1.5	112.5
Apple Berry	1	2	1.5	112.5
Chocolate Ck	1	2	1.5	112.5
Ft Boosters	1	2	1.8	135
Munchos	l oz	9	2	150
No Fri Rancho	1 oz.	2	1.5	112.5
No Fri Cheese Puff	1 oz.	2	1.5	112.5
Nuts:				
Miscellaneous	1 oz.	15	2.25	169
Peanuts	1 oz	14	2	150
Honey Rst Pea	1 oz.	13	2	150
In the Shell	1 oz.	14	2	150
Spanish peanuts	1 oz.	14	2.3	172.5
Sunflower Seed	1 oz.	15	2.3	172.5
Olives, green	3 lg/6 med	3.6	0.5	37.5
Olives, ripe	2 lg 6 sm	4	0.5	37.5
Pate'	1 oz.	3.7	0.7	52.5
Pickles:				
Dill Chips	24	0	.5	37.5
Dill Relish	2 T.	0	0	0

APPETIZERS (continued)

FOOD	AMOUNT	FAT GRAMS	CALORIE PTS	CALORIES
Pickles:				
Dill, Whole	4	0	0.5	37.5
Bread & Butter	8 slices	0	0.5	37.5
Sw Gherkins	4	0	0.5	37.5
Sweet Relish	2 T.	0	0.5	37.5
Popcorn, air pop	3 cups	1.4	1	75
Popcorn, oil	2 cups	4	1	75
Popcorn caramel	1 cup	1.5	1.5	112.5
Popcorn, Micrwv	3cups	5	1.3	97.5
Jolly Time,nat'l	3cups	5	1	75
Jolly Time, bt, nat'l	3 cups	1.8	1.3	97.5
Orville Red Gour	3 cups	5	1	75
Orville Light	3 cups	1	0.7	52.5
Pop Secret	3 cups	6	1.3	97.5
Pop Secret Lt	3 cups	3	1	75
Vic's popcorn	1 cup	4	.0.7	52.5
Vic's Lite	1 cup	3	2.7	202.5
Vic's Ched Lt	2.5 cups	7	1.9	142.5
Vic's Caramel	1 cup	6	3	225
Vic's Caramel lt	1 cup	2	1.5	112.5
Pork Skins	1/2 oz.	5	1	75
Pretzels Bked Super	1	0	1.5	112.5
Pretzels, Dutch	1 avg	0.6	1	75
Pretzels, x thin	75	1	1	75
Pretzels, Mustard	1 oz.	4	1.7	127.5
Pretzels 3 ring	3	0.6	1	75
Pretzels, Stick	35	0.5	1	75
Rtz Snk Mix Ch	1 oz.	6	1.75	131
Rtz Snk Mix Tr	1 oz.	6	1.75	131
Seeds, Shelled:				
Pistachio	2 T	0.7	1	75
Pumpkin	2 T.	7.9	1	75
Pumpkin, Dried	1 oz.	13	1.5	112.5
Sunflower	2 T.	8.8	1.2	90
Tortilla Rice Bte	1/2 oz.	0.5	0.7	52.5
Tostitos, Bk	1 oz. (13)	1	1.4	105
Tostitos, Bk Rnc	1 oz. (14)	3	1.6	120
T. Marzettis:				
Carmel ff apple	dip 2 T.	0	1.5	112.5
Choc ff banana	dip 2 T.	0	1.6	120

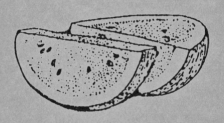

BEVERAGES

Balancing fluid intake today is hard for many people...either they have very little water, or fluids for the day, or they drink great quantities as fillers, as a caffeine buzz, as a habit, and may take in more calories than they've ever considered. A lady drinking 350 calories of juice per day that is beyond her calorie needs, can gain one pound every ten days.....

Work at increasing water, and then read through the next clue twice to see how it applies to you.

Karen's Klue: Drink one glass of water for every cup or glass of your favorite beverage, you will save calories, take care of thirst, and gradually reduce without deprivation the caffeine or sugar intake. Rule of thumb. We need one half of our body weight in water daily. (I.E. 130 pound female needs 65 oz. water daily-before activity)

BEVERAGES

FOOD	AMOUNT	FAT GRAMS	CALORIE PTS	CALORIES
Alcohol:				
Whiskey, Wine, Bourbon, Brandy,				
Scotch, Vodka				
Rum, Gin	1 oz.	0	1	75
Beer	12 oz.	0	2	150
Beer Lite	12 oz.	0	1.3	97.5
Wine, Sweet	3 1/2 oz.	0	2	150
Wine, table	3-4 oz.	0	1	75
AllSport	8 oz.	0	1	75
Diet Carn H. Cho	1 pkg	0	0.3	22.5
Carn Sugar Free	1 pkg	tr.	1	75
Rich Chocolate	1 pkg	1	1.5	112.5
70 Calorie	3 t.	tr.	1	75
S.F. Prem Coc	1 pkg	tr.	1	75
Clearly Canada	8 oz.	0	1.1	82.5
Club Soda	8 oz.	0	0	0
Cocoa Dry Mx	1 cup	3.1	1.3	97.5
Coffee	8 oz.	0	0	0
Crystal Light	8 oz..	0	0.1	7.5
Eggnog	8 oz.	19	3	225
Eggnog, alcohol	8 oz.	15.8	4	300
Free & clear	8 oz.	0	0	0
Frt Drnk, Sugar Su	8 oz.	0	0	0
Frt Drnk, 10% juice	8 oz	0	0.2	15
Fruit Juices	See Fruits			
Gatorade, Grape	8 oz.	0	0.7	52.5
Gatorade, other	8 oz.	0	1.6	120
Hi-C orange	8 oz.	0	1.7	127.5
Juicy Juice	8 oz	0	1.7	127.5
Lemonade	8 oz.	0	1	75
Lipton Diet Orig.	8 oz.	0	0	0
Lipton Peach	8 oz.	0	1.2	90
Milk	See Dairy Foods			
Nestle Quick,				
Sugar Free	2 T.	1	0.5	40
NY Seltzer flav.	10 oz.	0	1.5	112.5
NY Seltzer orig.	10 oz.	0	1.5	112.5
O. Spray cranch.	8 oz.	0	2.1	157.5
PoweAde, grape	8 oz.	0	1	75
Sam's chc. rasp	8 oz.	0	1.2	90
Snapple. strawb	8 oz.	0	1.7	127.5

BEVERAGES (continued)

FOOD	AMOUNT	FAT GRAMS	CALORIE PTS	CALORIES
Soda Pop	12 oz.	0	2	150
Soda Pop, diet	12 oz.	0	0	0
Squeezit, cherry	8 oz.	0	1.7	127.5
Squeezit, punch	8 oz.	0	1.4	105
Tang type mix	8 oz.	0	1.5	112.5
Tea	8 oz.	0	0	0
Tonic Water	8 oz.	0	1.5	112.5
V-8	8 oz.	tr.	0.5	37.5
Water	8 oz.	0	0	0

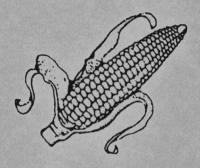

BREADS & GRAINS

Hearty and Healthy. . .All of you over 35 who were taught these were fattening need to read and study every work of knowledge on carbohydrates. We give you **Page 6 Concerning the Carb Craze**. The healthiest plans for lowering weight, cholesterol, blood sugar, and other health goals should include a diet rich in grains. As you can tell many of our breads and people's tastes are refined without fiber and chewiness, i.e. white bread. . . . You can see on the **Pyramid, Page 30** the number any of us can get per day for a healthy range. Breads are obviously low in fat, fill the stomach, and high in nutrients we need. Don't let the bulk fool you. When we increase breads and grains you may see some increase body water weight initially, but this is not bad or permanent, this is protective to save muscle.

Karen's Klue: One chewy slice of toast, a few crunchy crackers, or other grains with texture, may slow down your eating and give you enough fullness to control eating through a meal or snack.

BREADS & GRAINS

FOOD	AMOUNT	FAT GRAMS	CALORIE PTS	CALORIES
Azteca Salad Shell	1	12	2.7	202.5
Bread	1	1	1	75
Bagel, Average	1 whole	1.4	2	150
Bagel, Lenders Plain	1	1	2	150
Bagel , Blueberry	1	2	2.5	187.5
Bagel, Sarah Lee	1	1	3	225
Banana Bread	1 med sl.	2.5	1.6	120
Breads, other fruit	1 med sl.	2.5	1.6	120
Bialy Bread	1	0	1	75
Biscuit	1 2" or 1 oz.	4.5	1.3	97.5
Boboli Bread	1 small	7	4	300
Boboli Bread	l/4 lge	7	4	300
Branola Brand Bread				
Country Oat	1 slice	2	1.3	97.5
Hearty Wheat	1 slice	2	1.3	97.5
Bread Stuffing	l/2 cup	1	2.5	187.5
Bun	1 1-l/2 oz	2	1.5	112.5
Cornbread	1sm.square	7.3	2.5	187.5
Dinner Roll	1 medium	1	1.5	112.5
D'Italiano Bread (light)	2 slices	1.5	1.1	82.5
D'Italiano breadsticks	1	1.5	1.5	112.5
D'Italiano Pizza Crust	1/4 small	4	2	150
Doughnuts:				
Cake-plain	1 medium	5.8	1.5	112.5
Cake-iced	1 medium	6.5	2	150
Raised-plain	1 medium	8	1.5	112.5
Raised-with jelly	1 medium	8.8	3	225
English Muffins	1/2 muffin	0.6	1.1	82.5
Fillo Dough	1 oz.	0.4	1	75
Hard Roll	1	1.7	1	75
Hush Puppies	1 (2 oz.)	7	2	150
J.C. Garlic Breadsticks	1	9	1.75	131
J.C. Garlic Loaf	2 oz.	9	1.75	131
Less Brand Lites Buns	1	1	1	75
Muffin (corn, bran, fruit)	1 medium	4.3	2	150
Krusteaz apple muffin	1 medium	0	1.7	127.5
Krusteaz FF blueberry	1 medium	0	1.7	127.5
Betty Crocker BB	1 medium	0.5	1.7	127.5
Oroweatlite wh. wheat	1	0	0.5	37.5
Pepperidge Farm Breads:				
Cracked Wheat	1 slice	2	2	150
Family pumpernickel	1 slice	2	2	150

BREADS & GRAINS (continued)

FOOD	AMOUNT	FAT GRAMS	CALORIE PTS	CALORIES
Pepperidge Farm Breads:				
Honey Wheatberry,	1 slice	2	2	150
Multi-grain very thin	2 slices	1	1	75
Raisin w/cinnamon	1 slice	3	2	150
Whole Wheat very thin	2 slices	2	1	75
Pepperidge F.Party Rye	4 slices	1	1	75
Pepp. F. Sour D. Light	1 slice	0.3	0.6	45
Pepp F. 7 Grain Light	1 slice	0.3	0.6	45
Pillsbury Ref Cr. French	1" slice	1	1	75
Pillsbury Grand's Bisc	1	9	2.66	199.5
Pillsbury Hearty Gr. Wt	1	2	1.3	97.5
Pillsbury Bd Stick	1	2	1.3	97.5
Pillsbury Pipin Hot	1	2	1.3	97.5
Pillsbury Soft Breadstick	1	2	1.3	97.5
Pocket Bread	1 small	0	1	75
Pop Tarts, Frosted	1 pastry	5	2.5	187.5
Pop tarts, Unfrosted	1 pastry	6	2.5	187.5
Raisin Bread	1 slice	1.5	1	75
Rice Cakes	1	0	0.5	37.5
Roman Meal :				
Cracked Wheat	1 slice	tr	1	75
Honey Wtberry Lt	1 slice	tr	0.5	37.5
Oat	1 slice	1	1	75
Sandwich Bread	1 slice	tr	0.8	60
Seven Grain Lt	1 slice	tr	0.5	37.5
White	1 slice	tr	1	75
Sara Lee Original:				
Butter Croissant	1 petite	6	1.5	112.5
Sweet Roll, Plain	1 1/2 oz.	6.9	2	150
Sweet roll icing & filling	1 1/2 oz.	8.9	3	225
Taco Shell	1	2.2	1	75
Toaster Pastry, fsted	1	5	3	225
Tortilla	1 small	1	1	75
Wheat Germ	3 T.	2.25	1.5	112.5

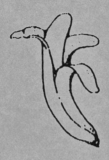

CANDY AND SWEETS

AHHHHHH. . . . .the sometimes foods. The guilt and the crazy eating styles today are filled with sugar. Americans averaged 134 pounds of granulated sugar in their diet last year - that is approximately 3/4 cup per day. . .and that's not good. Many people I work with make some guidelines/rules to control sweets, and for most of us that needs to be often enough to satisfy the craving, and our social life, yet not so frequently that they replace foods with real health value. One of my elderly clients, who will live long because of his knowledge and attitude calls these foods dead calories. . .When we think about the effects they should only be sometimes foods.

Work to get away from the sweetest tastes, to sweet flavors. Some of the products now that are sweetened with fruit or aspartame are excellent. You don't have to give up every family dessert. You may need to reduce the sugar in the recipe. The experts believe you can cut 1/3 minimum to 1/2 maximum and still have a quality, and great tasting product.

Karen's Klue: For every sweet or non-nutritive food, have a choice with real health value. (i.e. you have two cookies, than have a glass of milk, if you want two more, you will need to have one more healthy food each time. . .)

CANDY & SWEETS

FOOD	AMOUNT	FAT GRAMS	CALORIE PTS	CALORIES
Candy Bars:				
Bar None	l.5 oz.	14	3.3	247.5
Butter Finger	2.1 oz.	11	2.8	210
100 Grand Bar	1.5 oz.	8	2.7	202.5
Hershey M. Choc.	1.65 oz.	14	3.3	250
Kit Kat Wafer	1.65 oz.	13	3.3	250
Nestle Alpine w/alm.	1.25 oz.	13	2.6	200
Nestle Crunch	1.4 oz.	10	2.6	200
Oh Henry	2 oz.	10	3.3	250
Snickers	2.2 oz.	14	4	300
3 Muskateers	2.1 oz.	8	3.5	260
Caramels	4 avg	4	1.5	113
Chewing gum	5 sticks	0	0.5	38
Chewing gum				
Sugarfree	7 sticks	0	0.25	19
Chocolate	1 oz.	9	1.75	131
M&M's, Plain	50	10	3	225
M&M's, Peanut	25	12	3	225
Chocolate Kiss	7 individual	9	2	150
Fruit Topping	1 Tbs	0	0.5	40
Fudge	1 " square	3.4	1.5	113
Fun Size Bars:				
After 8 Mint	1	1	0.5	38
Alpine White	1	4	0.75	56
Baby Ruth	1	5	1.3	100
Chunky	1	4	1.3	100
Crunch	1	3	0.6	50
Grand	1	4	1.3	100
Heath	1	3	0.6	45
Kit Kat	1	4	1.1	82.5
Milk Chocolate	1	3	0.6	45
Milky Way	1	3.5	1.2	90
Oh Henry	1	3	0.8	60
Raisinets	1 pkg.	2	0.6	45
Snickers	1	4.5	1.3	97.5
3 Muskateers	1	2	1	75
Gumdrops	8 small	0	0.5	37.5
Gummy Bears	1 oz.	0	1.3	97.5
Hard Candy	1 oz.	0	1.5	112.5
Hersh Ckie&Mnt	1	4.5	1.1	82.5
Hugs/Almonds	1.4 oz.	14	3	225
Jam/Jelly	1 Tbsp	0	1	75
Diet Jelly	1 Tbsp	0	0.3	22.5

CANDY & SWEETS (continued)

FOOD	AMOUNT	FAT GRAMS	CALORIE PTS	CALORIES
Jelly Beans	10	0	1	75
Licorice	1.5 oz	0	2	150
Twizzlers	1 oz.	0	1.3	97.5
Cherry Nibs	1	0	1.3	97.5
Lifesavers	10	0	1	75
Lollipop	1	0	1	75
Marshmallows	1lge/1/3c.sm.	0	0.5	37.5
Malted Milk Ball	14	7	2	150
Peppermints	3	0.5	1	75
Choc Cr.De Menthe	4	0.5	1	75
Pastel Pillow Mint	6	0	1	75
Peanut Brittle	1 oz.	4.5	1.66	124.5
NutRageous	1	15	3.5	262.5
R. P. Butter Cup	1 cup	6	1.4	105
Sugarless Discs	1 oz.	0	0.5	37.5
Sugarless Sucker	1 sm	0	0.5	37.5
Taffy	1 1" cube	1.5	0.5	37.5
Twix	1 cookie	6	1.6	120
Werthers Orig.	3 pieces	1	1	75

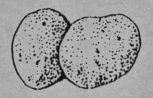

CEREALS

Much of what I've stated on breads and grains, and Concerning the Carb Craze, applies to cereal. Many people prefer this for snacks - not as traditional breakfast. This is a good time to remind you that sugar content really varies in cereal and you need to read the label. One teaspoon sugar is 5 grams. Some may have 30 grams in candy-like sweetened cereal. Other cereal is as wholesome and high in fiber and nutrients as any food available.

Karen's Klue: By combining a higher fiber, less sweet cereal with a small amount of granola may satisfy your craving just fine.

CEREALS

FOOD	AMOUNT	FAT GRAMS	CALORIE PTS	CALORIES
Cooked:				
Apple & Cinnamon	1 pkg	0	2	150
Brown Sugar	1 pkg	0	2	150
Maple	1 pkg	0	2	150
Plain	1 pkg	0	2	150
Peach & Strbrry	1 pkg	2	2	150
Malt O Meal	3/4 c.	0.5	1.3	97.5
Quaker Ins Oatmeal	1 pkg	2	1.8	135
Qker Multigrain	1/2 c. dry	1.5	1.8	135
Qker Oats + Fiber	l/2 c. dry	2.5	1.8	135
Qker Ots Raisin Br	1/2 c. dry	2	2	150
Ready to Eat:				
All-Bran, Kellogg	1/3 c	1	1	75
All-Bran Nabisco	1 oz.	1	1	75
Alpha Bits	1 c.	tr	1.5	112.5
Apple Jacks	1 oz.	0	1.3	97.5
Blueberry Mrng	1 1/4 c.	3.5	3.6	270
Bran Flakes	2/3 c	0	1	75
Captain Crunch	3/4 c.	3	1.5	112.5
Cheerios	3/4 c.	2	1.5	112.5
Chex	2/3 c.	0	1	75
Cinn. Mini Buns	3 1/2 oz.	2	5	375
Cinn. Toast Crunch	1 c.	3	1.5	112.5
Cocoa Krispies	3/4 c.	0	1.5	112.5
Cocoa Puffs	1 c.	1	1.5	112.5
Cmplt Bran Flks	3/4 oz	0	1	75
Cornflakes	1 c.	0	1.3	97.5
Corn Pops	1 c.	0	1.5	112.5
Cracklin Oat Brn	3 1/2 oz	12	5	375
Crispex	1 c.	0	1.5	112.5
Crispy Critters	1 c.	tr	1.5	112.5
Fruit Loops	1 c.	1	1.5	112.5
Frosted Bran	1 oz	0	1.3	97.5
Frosted Flakes	3/4 c.	0	1.5	112.5
Frosted Min. Wts	4 bsc.	0	1.5	112.5
Fruit and Fiber	1/2 c	1	1	75
Golden Grams	3/4 c.	1	1.5	112.5
Granola bars	See convenience			
Grape Nuts	1/4 c	0	1.3	97.5
Grape Nut Flake	1 c.	0	1.5	112.5

CEREALS (continued)

FOOD	AMOUNT	FAT GRAMS	CALORIE PTS	CALORIES
Health Valley:				
Cinnamon O's	1 oz.	1	1.3	97.5
High Fibers O's	1 oz.	1	1.3	97.5
H. Nut Cheerios	1 c.	1	1.5	112.5
Just Right	2 oz.	2	2	150
Kell. Raisin Bran	2/3 c.	1	1.7	127.5
Kell. Raisin. Nut Bran	2/3 c.	3	1.5	112.5
Kell. L. Fat Granola	1.5 oz.	3	2	150
Lucky Charms	1 c.	1	1.5	112.5
Muselix Bran	1/2 c	2	1.8	135
Natl Raisin Bran	1/2 c	0	1	75
Nectar Oat Bran	1 oz.	5	1.5	112.5
Nut & Honey Crunch	1 oz.	1	1.8	135
Post Oat Flakes	2/3 c	tr	1.5	112.5
Post Raisin Bran	2/3 c	1	1.7	127.5
Product 19	1 c.	0	1.3	97.5
Puffed Rice	1 c.	0	0.5	37.5
Puffed Wheat	1 c.	0	0.5	37.5
Rice Crispies	1 c.	0	1.5	112.5
Shredded Wheat	1 bsc	tr	1	75
Smacks	1 oz.	0	1.7	127.5
Special K	1 c.	0	1.5	112.5
Total	1 c.	0	1.5	112.5
Trix	1 c.	1	1.5	112.5
Wheaties	1 c.	1	1.5	112.5

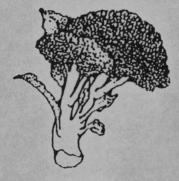

CHEESE

Today low fat diets don't have to suffer without cheese, or cheese that tastes good. First measure out an ounce so you know what your portion really is. All of us who love cheese could consume several ounces when we've sworn that it wasn't much... There are all kinds of cheese out there containing low to no fat content. Larger stores and larger cities tend to carry more of these products, probably due to the numbers who've experimented and found good-tasting products and come back for more.

If nothing else, mix regular and lite cheese. Decrease amounts in entrees and casseroles, by shredding and sprinkling, not slicing or covering. Cheese spreads may help in saving you fat grams as well, due to increased carbohydrates (flours etc.) and great melting ability.

Karen's Klue - Kraft's Healthy Favorites Fat Free Cheddar or Mozzarella are great tasting shredded cheese that melt on a tortilla or sandwich. Look for the red label. When available the low fat versions may work better in entrees etc....

CHEESE

FOOD	AMOUNT	FAT GRAMS	CALORIE PTS	CALORIES
AMERICAN:				
Alpine lace	1 oz.	0	0.3	22.5
Borden Lite Line	1 oz.	0	0.5	37.5
Borden Lt Low Chol	1 oz.	7	1.25	94
Healthy Choice	1 slice	0	0.5	37.5
Healthy Favorite	1 slice	2	0.6	45
Healthy Favorite	1 oz.	3	0.8	60
Kraft Free Slices	1 oz.	0.7	0.7	52.5
Kraft Lt and Lively	1 oz.	4	1	75
Velveeta	1 oz.	6	1	75
Velveeta Italian	1 oz.	6	1	75
Velveeta Light	1 oz.	3	0.66	49.5
Velveeta Lt Singles	1 oz.	4	1	75
Weight Watchers	1 oz.	1	0.5	37.5
World's Fare				
Lite 'n Low	1 oz.	6	1	75
BLUE:				
Blue Spread, Roka	1 oz.	6	1	75
Kraft	1 oz.	9	1.3	97.5
Sargento	1 oz.	8	1.3	97.5
CHEDDAR:				
Alpine Lace				
Low Sod.	1 oz	8	1.3	97.5
Healthy Choice				
Cheddar	1 oz.	0	0.5	37.5
Lt Healthy Choice	1 oz.	4	1	75
Kraft Free Sharp	1 oz.	0	0.7	52.5
Kraft Light Natural	1 oz.	5	1	75
Wt Watchers				
40% less fat	1 oz.	5	1	75
World's Fare				
Lt Cheddar	1 oz.	8	1	75
COLBY:				
Alpine Lace				
Low Sod.	1 oz.	5	1	75
Healthy Fav Colby	1 oz.	4	1	75
Healthy Choice	1 oz.	0	0.5	37.5
Kraft Natural				
Red. Fat	1 oz.	5	1	75
Worlds Fare				
Lt Colby	1 oz.	5	1	75

CHEESE (continued)

FOOD	AMOUNT	FAT GRAMS	CALORIE PTS	CALORIES
COTTAGE CHEESE:				
Creamed	l/2 cup	5	1.5	112.5
Dry curd	l/2 cup	0.3	1.5	112.5
Low fat, 2%	1/2 cup	2	1.3	97.5
Viva Fat Free	l/2 cup	0	0.8	60
CREAM CHEESE:				0
Healthy Choice	1 oz.	0	0.5	37.5
Kraft Healthy				
Favorites	1 oz.	5	0.75	56.25
Philly Reduce Fat	1 oz.	5	1	75
Philly Free	1 oz.	0	0.5	37.5
Wt Watchers	1 oz.	2	0.5	37.5
MONTEREY JACK:				0
Alpine Lace Low				
Sodium	1 oz.	4	1	75
Kraft Healthy				
Favorites	1 oz.	4	1	75
Kraft Natural				
Reduced Fat	1 oz.	5	1	75
Wt Watchers	1 oz.	5	1	75
MOZZARELLA:				
Part skim	1 oz.	5	1	75
Alpine Lace Low				
Sodium	1 oz.	4	1	75
Healthy Choice Ball	1 oz.	0	0.5	37.5
Kraft	1 oz.	5	1	75
Kraft Healthy				
Favorites	1 oz.	3	0.8	60
NEUFCHATEL:				
Light, Philly	1 oz.	7	1	75
PARMESAN:				
Kraft, grated	1 oz.	9	1.8	135
Kraft, Natural	1 oz.	7	1.5	112.5
Sargento, fresh	1 oz.	7	1.5	112.5
Sargento Parmesan				
and Romano Grated	1 oz.	7	1.5	112.5
PROCESSED SPREAD:				
Cheese Whiz				
All varieties	1 oz.	6	1	75
Cheese Whiz, Lt	1 oz.	3	1	75

CHEESE (continued)

FOOD	AMOUNT	FAT GRAMS	CALORIE PTS	CALORIES
Kraft Flavored				
Spreads	1 oz.	5	1	75
Old Eng Cheese				
Sprd	1 oz.	7	1	75
Squeeze a Snak	1 oz.	7	1	75
RICOTTA:				
Whole Milk	1 oz.	16	3	225
Part Skim	1 oz.	2	2.3	172.5
STRING CHEESE:				
Healthy Choice	1 oz.	0	0.5	37.5
Kraft l00% Part Skim	1 oz.	5	1	75
Sargento	1 oz.	5	1	75
SWISS:				
Alpine Swiss Low				
Sodium	1 oz.	6	1.3	97.5
Borden Lt Line	1 oz.	2	0.7	52.5
Kraft Free	1 oz.	0	0.66	49.5
Kraft Healthy				
Favorites	1 oz.	4	1	75
Kraft Lt and Lively	1 oz.	3	1	75
Worlds Fare				
Lt & Low	1 oz.	7	1.3	97.5
MISCELLANEOUS				
CHEESE PRODUCTS:				
Alpine Cheese Hot				
Pepper	1 oz.	6	1	75
Cracker Barrel				
Cheese Logs	1oz.	6	1	75
Easy Cheese				
All Varieties	1 oz.	6	1	75
Feta Cheese	1 oz.	8	1	75
Handi Snaks Cz &				
Crackers	1 pkg	8	1.5	112.5
Handi Snaks P.B.				
& Cheez	1 pkg	14	2.5	187.5
World's Fare				
Muenster	1 oz.	8	1.3	97.5

DIETARY GUIDELINES

- Eat a variety of foods

- Balance the food you eat with physical activity-maintain or improve your weight

- Choose a diet with plenty of grain products, vegetables, and fruits

- Choose a diet low in saturated fat and cholesterol

- Choose a diet moderate in sugars

- Choose a diet moderate in salt and sodium

- If you drink alcoholic beverages, do so in moderation

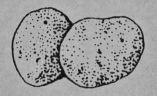

CHIPS

When studying chips, you may want to go back to appetizers for other crunchy foods that may fit your need to chew. Another rule of thumb is eating two or three other nutritive choices with the chips and limiting the bag size. One ounce bags for sack lunches, or a snack, satisfies the initial taste, and yet leaves you with no regrets and high fat intakes. The final work is not in on olestra products and people's ability to modify and comfortably digest. Yet with all the baked products, you have a choice with no real issues, and taste that keeps improving.

Karen's Klue: Try the baked tostito's with fat free refried bean appetizer, garnished with fat free or low fat cheese, fat free sour cream, and spicy salsa. Your friends may not even know. . . .

CHIPS

FOOD	AMOUNT	FAT GRAMS	CALORIE PTS	CALORIES
Cheetos Light	appr. 34 pcs.	6	1.5	112.5
Doritos	1 oz.	6	2	150
Doritos, flavored	1 oz.	7	2	150
Doritos Light, Nacho	15 chips	4	1.5	112.5
LOUISE'S POT. CHIPS				
Original	1 oz.	<1	1.3	97.5
Maui Onion	1 oz.	<1	1.3	97.5
Mesquite Barbecue	1 oz.	<1	1.3	97.5
Mr. Phipps Tortilla Chips	29 chips	4.5	1.8	135
PACIFIC GRAIN POT. C				
Barbecue	30 pieces	1.5	1.8	135
Cheddar Jalapeno	30 pieces	2	1.8	135
Salsa &Sour Cream	30 pieces	2	1.8	135
Sour Cream & Chives	30 pieces	2	1.8	135
POPSECRET P. CHIPS				
Original	1 1/2 cups	3.5	1.8	135
Butter	1 1/2 cups	3.5	1.8	135
Sour Cream & Onion	1 1/2 cups	3.5	1.8	135
Potato Chips	1 oz.	10	2.5	187.5
Potato Chips	7 chips	4	1	75
PRINGLES				
Potato chips	18	12	2.3	172.5
Corn chips	11	7	2	150
Light Variety	20	8	2	150
Ruffles Light Potato Chip	18	6	1.5	112.5
Tostitos Chips, baked	1 oz. (13)	1	1.4	105
Tostitos baked ranch	1 oz. (14)	3	1.5	112.5
Lays baked	1 oz.	1.5	1.5	112.5
Lays baked, ranch	1 oz.	1.5	1.5	112.5

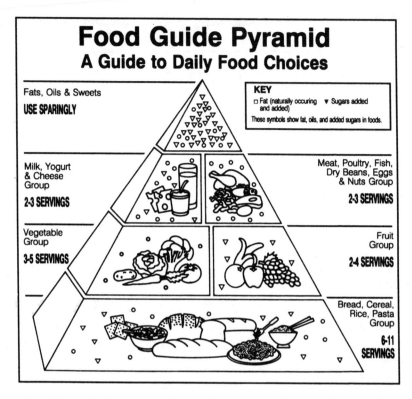

Food Guide Pyramid
A Guide to Daily Food Choices

Fats, Oils & Sweets
USE SPARINGLY

Milk, Yogurt
& Cheese
Group
2-3 SERVINGS

Meat, Poultry, Fish,
Dry Beans, Eggs
& Nuts Group
2-3 SERVINGS

Vegetable
Group
3-5 SERVINGS

Fruit
Group
2-4 SERVINGS

Bread, Cereal,
Rice, Pasta
Group
**6-11
SERVINGS**

The **Food Guide Pyramid** emphasizes foods from the five food groups shown in the three lower sections of the Pyramid.

Each of these food groups provides some, but not all, of the nutrients you need. Foods in one group can't replace those in another. No one food group is more important than another - or good health, you need them all.

The Pyramid is an outline of what to eat each day. It's not a rigid prescription, but a general guide that lets you choose a healthful diet that's right for you. The pyramid calls for eating a variety of foods to get the nutrients you need and at the same time the right amount of calories to maintain a healthy weight.

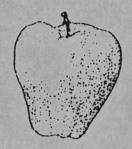

CONVENIENCE FOODS

Today's population has much to learn abut the products that save us time and labor. We get more fat in this area than meat and milk, if we ignore labels and ingredients. Yet the food choices with nutritional advantages are there, if you've done your homework. If you study this area before the grocery store shopping and have a few items on hand, it will save you a great deal of calories and fat. Even those who have time and desires to cook homemade products usually benefit if they have some convenience items on hand. Sodium content is an issue only if you don't know milligrams and recommendations for all of us is 24000 mg/day, while many Americans take in 6-8000 milligrams. Do you add less than 1/4 teaspoon to some foods. . . .Check and find out.

Karen's Klue: Have a few favorite entrees on hand and add your own side dishes, for a meal prepared in under ten minutes, and yet economical with variety in nutrients and tastes (i.e. my chicken rice/vegetable light entree is great with toast and fresh grapes).

CONVENIENCE FOODS

FOOD	AMOUNT	FAT GRAMS	CALORIE PTS	CALORIES
BREAKFAST FOODS				
AUNT JAMIMA:				
Orig. Pancake & W Mix	3-4"ckes	8	3	225
Buttermilk Mix	3-4"ckes	11	4	300
Complete Mix	3-4"ckes	4	4	300
Complete Buttermilk	3-4"ckes	3	3	225
Butter Lt Syrup	1 oz.	0	0.7	49.5
Lt Syrup	1 oz.	0	0.8	60
Syrup	1 oz.	0	0.8	60
Betty Crock Wild Blue B				
Muffin Mix	1	0.5	1.7	127.5
Carnation Brk Bar, Cho C	1	11	2.3	172.5
Carn Instant Brkfst	1 pkg	tr	1.7	127.5
Carn Inst. Brkfst SF	1 pkg	tr	1	75
Healthy Valley Brkfst Bar				
Chocolate	1	0	1.5	112.5
Fruit Fitness	1	0	1.5	112.5
Strawberry	1	0	2	150
Hostess Brkfst				
Apple Streusel Muffin	1	1	1.3	97.5
Blueberry Muffin	1	2	1.3	97.5
Snackwell FF Cereal b	1	0	1.5	112.5
GRANOLA BARS:				
Amer Fit. Classics	1	0	1.6	120
Archway Bar	1	0	1	75
Betty Crocker Inc. Bites	1	8	2.3	172.5
Flavor Kist Pastry Bar	1	3	1.8	135
Kelloggs LF Bar	1	2	1	75
Kudo's Snacks	1	12	2.7	202.5
Nature Valley, All Variet	1	5	1.7	127.5
Nature Valley LF	1	2	1.4	105
Nutra Grain Cereal	1	5	2	150
Quaker Chewy LF Bar				
Apple Berry	1	2	1.5	112.5
Choc. Chunk	1	2	1.5	112.5
Sunbelt Ft Boosters	1	2	1.8	135
CHINESE:				
Eggroll	1	10	1.5	112.5
Fortune Cookies	2	0	0.5	37.5
Fried Rice	1 cup	15	2.5	187.5
LaChoy:				
Vegetable, Variety	1/2 cup	0.1	0.3	22.5
Beef Chow Mein	3/4 cup	2	3.3	247.5

CONVENIENCE FOODS (continued)

FOOD	AMOUNT	FAT GRAMS	CALORIE PTS	CALORIES
Chinese Food (continued):				
Beef Pepper Entree	3/4 cup	4	1.3	97.5
Chicken Chow Mein	3/4 cup	4	1	75
Chicken Chow Mein Dn	l/2 pkg	17	4	300
Chow Mein Noodles	l/2 cup	8	2	150
Fried Rice	3/4 cup	1	2.5	187.5
Meatless Chow Mein	3/4 cup	1	2.5	187.5
Shrimp Chow Mein	3/4 cup	17	4	300
Sw & Sr Chicken	3/4 cup	2	3.3	247.5
FROZEN:				
BREAKFAST FOODS				
Healthy Choice:				
Blueberry Muffins	1	4	2.5	187.5
Eng. Muff Sandwich	1	3	2.3	172.5
Western Omelet w/ muff	1	3	2.3	172.5
Krusteaz Fr. Toast	1	3	1.5	112.5
Krusteaz Pancakes	3	5	3.8	285
Krusteaz B.B. Pancake	3	5	4	300
Swanson Great Starts				
Bel Waffle w/ Strbrry S.	1 pkg	7	2.8	210
Bacon Burrito	1	11	3.3	247.5
Eng muffin Bacon egg	1 pkg	16	4	300
Eng muff Sausage egg	1 pkg	29	6	450
Farmrich Fr. Tst Sticks	4	14	4	300
Pillsbury Toaster Strudel	1	9	2.3	172.5
WAFFLES:				
A. Jamima Blueberry	1	3	1	75
A. Jamima Homestyle	1	3	1	75
Belgium Chef	1	3	1	75
Downy Flake Blueberry	1	2	1	75
Downy Flake Buttermilk	1	2	1	75
Eggo Blueberry	1	5	1.8	135
Eggo Buttermilk	1	5	1.5	112.5
Eggo Homestyle	1	5	1.5	112.5
Eggo Nut & Honey	1	5	1.8	135
Eggo Special K	1	0	1	75
Jimmy D. Blueberry	1	10	1.5	112.5
Jimmy D. Flapsticks	1	12	2.3	172.5
WEIGHT WATCHERS:				
Apple Sweetrolls	1	3	2	150
Ham & Chz Bagel	1	6	2.8	210
Multi Grain Waffle	1	4	2.8	210
Sausage Biscuit	1	11	3	225

CONVENIENCE FOODS (continued)

FOOD	AMOUNT	FAT GRAMS	CALORIE PTS	CALORIES
BIRDS EYE EASY RECIPE:				
Beef Oriental	3.5 oz.	7	1.8	135
BUDGET GOURMET LT:				
Beef Stroganoff	1	12	4	300
Cheese Lasagna & Veg	1	9	4	300
Chicken Au Gratin	1	11	3.3	247.5
Ham & Asparagus Au Gr.	1	12	4	300
Linquini w/scllps & clams	1	11	4	300
Sirloin of beef	1	10	4	300
Turkey w/herb gravy	1	8	4	300
Teriyaki chicken	1	9	3.5	262.5
CAFE PASTA:				
Beef Tortelloni	1 oz. (10)	1.8	1	75
Cheese Tortelloni	1 oz. (8)	1.5	1	75
Jumbo Beef Ravioli	1	1.5	0.8	60
Jumbo Cheese Ravioli	1	2.8	0.8	60
Swanson Chckn Alaking	5.3	12	2.5	187.5
Swanson Chckn & Dump.	7.5	12	3	225
CHICKEN PRODUCTS:				
Banquet Fried chckn	6.4 oz.	19	4.3	322.5
Banquet Fried. br.portion	5.8 oz.	11	3	225
Bnqu. hot & spicy breast	2.3 oz.	6	2	150
Bnqu. hot bite chckn nug	2.5 oz.	14	3	225
Butterball turkey br. slice	1.4 oz.	1	1.5	112.5
Country Pride chicken chunks	3 oz.	15	3.8	285
CP South fried chicken patties	3 oz.	15	4.5	337.5
Weight Watch chck nug	4 nuggets	11	2.5	187.5
TYSON CHICKEN PRODUCTS:				
BBQ Breast Fillet	3 oz.	3	1.3	97.5
Breast Chunks	3 oz.	17	3.3	247.5
Breast Fillets	3oz.	9	2.5	187.5
Breast Patties	2.6 oz.	15	3.5	262.5
Chicken Pie	9 oz.	20	5.3	397.5
Diced Chicken Meat	3 oz.	3	1.8	135
Fajita Kit	3.5 oz.	5	2	150
Grilled Breast Fillet	2.8 oz.	3	1.3	97.5
Grilled Breast Tenders	2.8 oz.	3	1.3	97.5
Grilled Chick. Sandwich	3.5 oz	5	2.7	202.5
Hot & Spicy Tenders	2.8 oz	3	1.3	97.5
Lemon Pepper Br.	2.8 oz	3	1.3	97.5
Mesquite Breast Ten	2.8 oz.	3	1.3	97.5

CONVENIENCE FOODS (continued)

FOOD	AMOUNT	FAT GRAMS	CALORIE PTS	CALORIES
TYSON CHICKEN PROD. (continued):				
BBQ Chicken Sand	4 oz.	6	3	225
Micro Tenders	3.5 oz	11	3	225
Oriental Brst Tenders	2.8 oz.	3	1.3	97.5
Southern Fried Br.	3 oz.	11	3	225
Stir Fry Kit	4 oz.	7	2.5	187.5
Turkey Pie	9 oz.	18	5	375
FROZEN FISH:				
Fisher Boy Fish Sticks	3 stks	5	1.7	127.5
Gorton's Fried Clam Stp	1/2 pkg	23	4	300
Mrs Pauls Cajun Style	10.5 oz	4	2.5	187.5
Mrs Pauls Fried Shrimp	3oz.	11	2.3	172.5
MRS PAULS HEALTHY TREASURE:				
Bd Fish Fillets	4 oz.	3	2.2	165
Bd Fish Sticks	2.5 oz	3	2.2	165
Light Fillets n Sauce	4.1 oz	3	1.4	105
HEALTHY CHOICE:				
BBQ Chicken	1	6	4.75	356
Beef Enchilada Dinner	1	7	4.8	360
Beef Pepper Steak	1	3	2.8	210
Fettucini Alfredo	1	7	3.3	247.5
Fish Fillet	1	4	1.8	135
Fish Sticks	1	4	1.5	112.5
Linguini w/ Shrimp	1	2	3	225
Macaroni and Cheese	1	6	3.8	285
Mesquite Chicken Din.	1	4	4.8	360
Salsa Chicken Dinner	1	2	3.3	247.5
Seafood Newburg	1	3	2.8	210
Shrimp Marinara	1	4	4	300
Sole w/Lemon Butter	1	4	4	300
Sweet and Sour Chicken	1	4	4	300
Turkey Dinner	1	3	3.5	262.5
LEAN CUISINE:				
Beef & Bean Enchilada	1	10	3.8	285
Chicken Enchilada	1	9	3.5	262.5
Chicken Fettucine	1	6	3.8	285
Extra Ch French Bd	1	12	4.8	360
Fiesta Chicken	1	6	3.3	247.5
Homestyle Turkey	1	3	4	300
Macaroni & Cheese	1	9	4	300
Zucchini Lasagna	1	7	3.5	262.5

CONVENIENCE FOODS (continued)

FOOD	AMOUNT	FAT GRAMS	CALORIE PTS	CALORIES
LE MENU LIGHT STYLE:				
Glazed Turkey	1	6	3.5	262.5
Salisbury Steak	1	7	3	225
Swedish Meatballs	1	8	3.5	262.5
Veal Marsala	1	6	3.5	262.5
OLD EL PASO:				
Chicken Chimichanga	1	20	3.25	244
Chicken Enchilada Din.	1 pkg	18	6	450
Chicken Ch Enchilada	1 entree	12	3	225
Chicken Sour Cr. Ench.	1 entree	19	3.8	285
PIZZA, HEALTHY CHOICE:				
Cheese	5.6 oz.	4	4.1	307.5
Pepperoni	6 oz.	9	4.8	360
Supreme	6.35 oz.	6	4.5	337.5
PIZZA, PAPPALO'S:				
3 Cheese	1/4 pizza	11	4.66	349.5
Pepperoni	1/4 pizza	9	5	375
Sausage, Pan	I/5 pizza	13	4.66	349.5
PIZZA, TOMBSTONE:				
Pepperoni Lt	1/2 pizza	10	3.5	262.5
Sausage Lt	I/2 pizza	8	3.3	247.5
Vegetable Lt	I/2 pizza	8	3.3	247.5
PIZZA, TOTINO'S:				
Canadian Bacon I0 oz.	1/2 pizza	13	4.7	352.5
Hamburger 10 oz.	1/2 pizza	17	4.7	352.5
Pepperoni 10 oz.	1/2 pizza	13	5	375
WEIGHT WATCHERS:				
Deluxe	1	9	4.3	322.5
Pepperoni	1	8	4.3	322.5
POTPIES:				
Banquet Beef	7 oz.	29	6	450
Banquet Chicken	7 oz.	27	6	450
Banquet Chunky Beef	10 oz.	29	7.3	547.5
Banquet Chunky Turkey	10 oz.	31	7.3	547.5
Banquet Macaroni & Ch	7 oz.	9	3	225
FROZEN VEGETABLES:				
BIRDS EYE:				
Bav. Style Vegetable	1/3 pkg	3	1	75
Broc. Caul & Cheese	4.8 oz.	4	1	75
Broccoli w/Cheese	5 oz.	5	1.5	112.5
Cauliflower w/Cheese	5 oz.	5	1.3	97.5
Fr. Green Beans	3 oz.	3	0.5	37.5

CONVENIENCE FOODS (continued)

FOOD	AMOUNT	FAT GRAMS	CALORIE PTS	CALORIES
Birds Eye (continued):				
Rice Broccoli AuGratin	5 oz.	4	2	150
Stir F. Vegetables	3.3 oz.	0	0.5	37.5
GREEN GIANT:				
Broccoli w/ cheese	1/2cup	2	0.8	60
Caul. w/ cheese	1/2 cup	2	0.8	60
Niblet Corn w/butter	1/2 cup	2	1.3	97.5
Pasta Accents	1/2 cup	4	1.3	97.5
Peas & Potatoes w/Sc	5 oz.	3	1.33	100
ORE IDA POTATOES:				
Cheddar Browns	3 oz.	2	1.3	97.5
Cottage Fries	3 oz.	5	1.5	112.5
Crinkle Cut Lights	3 oz.	2	1.3	97.5
Crispers	3 oz.	15	3	225
Golden Crinkles	3 oz.	4	1.5	112.5
Hash Browns, Shred	3 oz.	tr	1.5	112.5
O'Brien Potatoes	3 oz.	tr	1	75
Pixie Crinkles	3 oz.	6	2	150
Shoestrings	3 oz.	6	2	150
Tator Tots	3 oz.	7	2	150
SCHWANS MEATS:				
Beef Fajita	3.5 oz	6	2	150
Beef Patty Melt	4 oz.	28	4.5	337.5
Chopped BB Beef	l/2 cup	8	2.9	217.5
Cr. Chipped Beef	3.5 oz	7	2	150
Lean Beef Patty	3.5 oz	11	2.4	180
Old Fashioned Weiners	2 oz.	16	2	150
Phili Style Beef Sandw.	3 sl	5	1.8	135
Pizza Patties	3.5 oz	22	3.5	262.5
Skinless Franks	1.6 oz	13	2	150
Sliced BBQ Beef Brisk	3.5 oz	5	2	150
Summer Sausage	2 oz.	13	2.1	157.5
BREADED MEATS:				
Breaded Cubed Beef	4 oz.	20	2.4	180
Breaded Steak Fingers	3.5 oz.	7	3	225
Center Cut Pork Loin	1 chip	5	1.8	135
Boneless Turkey Br w/Gravy	3.5 oz.	5	1.5	112.5
Breaded Chicken Brst Strips	3.5 oz.	14	3.5	262.5
Chicken Cordon Blue	5 oz.	14	4	300
Chicken Fajita	3.5 oz	2	1.5	112.5
Chicken Kiev	1	21	4.6	345

CONVENIENCE FOODS (continued)

FOOD	AMOUNT	FAT GRAMS	CALORIE PTS	CALORIES
SCHWANS MEATS (continued):				
Ht & Spicy Chicken Nug	3.5 oz	19	4.25	319
Hot Wings	3.5 oz	14	3	225
Southern Style Chick Fi	3.5 oz	11	2.75	206
Turkey Roll	3.5 oz.	7	2	150
Unbreaded Chicken Br	3.3 oz.	1	1.25	94
Unbreaded Turkey fillet	3 oz.	0	1	75
FAMILY ENTREE:				
Beef Ravioli	3.5 oz	4	2.5	187.5
Beef Teriyaki	11 oz.	14	5.8	435
Cheese Tortillini	3.5 oz.	5	3	225
Chicken Casserole	3.5 oz	8	2	150
Cr. of Broccoli Soup	1 cup	10	2.4	180
Homestyle Beef Goula	1 cup	13	3.7	277.5
Lasagna w/ Mt Sauce	3.5 oz	6	2	150
Shrimp Oriental	10 oz.	3	2.5	187.5
Stuffed Pasta Shells	2 oz. (1)	5	1.75	131
Wisconsin Cheese Soup	8 oz.	6	3	225
FISH FILLETS:				
Cod Fillets	3.5 oz.	0.5	1.2	90
Halibut Steaks	3.5 oz.	2	1.5	112.5
Ocean Perch	4 oz.	2	1.2	90
Orange Roughy	4 oz.	1.5	1.1	82.5
Red Snapper	3.5 oz.	1	1.3	99.8
BREADED SEAFOOD:				
Batter Crisp Cod	2 oz.	8	2	150
Breaded Fantail Shrimp	4 pc	1.5	2.2	165
Catfish Fingers	3.5 oz	13	3	225
Cod Fish Nuggets	3.5 oz	10	2.66	199.5
Oven Ready Bd Shrimp	3.5 oz	13	3.5	262.5
Stuffed Shrimp	2 oz.	7	1.8	135
Stuffed Sole Monterey	5 oz.	8	2.3	172.5
PREMIUM PORK PRODUCTS:				
Haugins Far Ham	3.5 oz	5	1.5	112.5
Pork Spare Ribs	3.5 oz	13	3.5	262.5
Sliced ham	1-1 oz. slice	2	0.5	37.5
PREMIUM STEAKS:				
Big Sam Steak	6 oz	18	4	300
Ribeye Steak	8 oz.	64	10	750
Sirloin Fillet of Beef	4 oz.	12	2.8	210
Tenderloin Steak	6 oz.	41	6.8	510

CONVENIENCE FOODS (continued)

FOOD	AMOUNT	FAT GRAMS	CALORIE PTS	CALORIES
SPECIAL RECIPE PIZZA:				
Canadian Style Bacon	3.5 oz.	14	3.8	285
Cheese	1/3 pizza	24	5.7	427.5
Hamburger	1/3 pizza	20	4.6	345
Sausage	3.5 oz	15	3.8	285
Supreme	3.5 oz.	16	3.8	285
Single Serve Pizza:				
Sausage	6 oz.	27	7.5	562.5
Supreme	6 oz.	29	8	600
ETHNIC FOODS:				
Apple Flautas	2 oz. (1)	3	2	150
Beef Chimichanga	5.8 oz. (1)	17	5	375
Brt Start Brkfst Burrito	1	17	3.7	277.5
Burritos	1	14	3.7	277.5
Cherry Flautas	2 oz. (1)	5	2	150
Shrimp Egg Rolls	2 pc.	4.5	2.4	180
Sanchos	5.8 oz. (1)	11	2.5	187.5
SANDWICHES:				
Bagel Dog w/Cheese	4.5 oz. (1)	21	5.5	412.5
Club Croissant	1	19	4.1	307.5
Ham Steak'n Egg Muff	4.3 oz. (1)	9	3.3	250
Rst Beef n-Swiss Crois	4.5 oz.	20	5	375
Sausage & Biscuit	1.6 oz.	11	2.5	187.5
FROZEN FRUIT & VEGETABLES:				
Breaded Onion Rings	3.5 oz.	14	3.5	262.5
Chunk Pineapple	3.5 oz.	<1	0.5	37.5
Corn on the Cob	9 oz. (1)	1	2.5	187.5
Crinkle Cut French Fries	3 oz. (27 pcs)	4	1.6	120
Italian Pasta Blend	3.5 oz.	1	0.8	60
Mixed Fruit	3.5 oz.	<1	0.5	37.5
Pierogies	1.3 oz.	1	1	75
Sliced Peaches	3.5 oz.	<1	0.5	37.5
Summer Garden Pasta	3.5 oz.	0	1	75
MISCELLANEOUS:				
Breaded Mozz. Sticks	2 sticks	6	1.3	97.5
Cinnamon rolls w/ icing	1	4.5	3.2	240
Frozen Bread Dough	2 oz.	1	2	150
Natural Lt MW Popcorn	3 T.	5	1.7	127.5
Stoneground Wheat Bread Dough	2 oz.	2	2	150
Waffles	3/4 oz.	6	1.3	97.5

CONVENIENCE FOODS (continued)

FOOD	AMOUNT	FAT GRAMS	CALORIE PTS	CALORIES
FROZEN TREATS:				
Chocolate Sundae Bar	1	8	2	150
Chocolate Caramel Nut	1	14	3.2	240
Fudge Stick	1	1	1.5	112.5
Golden' Nugget Bar	1	16	3.3	247.5
Ice Cream Sandwiches	1	6	2	150
Orange Pushups	1	<1	1	75
Pecan Praline Sun.	1	12	3.5	262.5
Schwan's Bar	1	14	2.8	210
Strawberry Yogurt Sand	1	4	2	150
Sundae Cup Cho. Malt	1	11	5.3	397.5
ICE CREAM:	1			
Black Raspberry	I/2 cup	7	2	150
Butter Pecan	I/2 cup	9	2	150
Cherry Vanilla	I/2 cup	7	2	150
Chip & Mint	I/2 cup	8	2	150
Chocolate Chips	I/2 cup	8	2	150
Chunky Choc Supreme	I/2 cup	9	2	150
Fresh Peach	I/2 cup	6	2	150
Rainbow Sherbet	I/2 cup	1	1.5	112.5
Raspberry Delight	I/2 cup	5	2	150
Summer's Dream	I/2 cup	5	2	150
Lite	I/2 cup	3	1.5	112.5
Extra lite Van & Strberry	I/2 cup	0	1.4	105
FROZEN YOGURT:				
Black Cherry	I/2 cup	2.5	1.6	120
Chocolate	I/2 cup	3	1.6	120
Vanilla	I/2 cup	3	1.4	105
MICROWAVE ENTREE:				
Beef Ravioli w/tomato sc	7.5 oz.	11	3	225
Dinty Moore Bf Stew	7.5 oz.	9	2.5	187.5
Hot Chili w/ Beans	7.5 oz.	11	3.3	247.5
Macaroni & Cheese	7.5 oz.	6	2.5	187.5
KRAFT:				
Beef Strog & Noodles	9 oz.	13	4.5	337.5
Chicken Cacciatore	10 oz.	6	3.5	262.5
Salsbury Steak	9.5 oz.	13	4	300
LIBBYS:				
Beans w/ Franks	7.75 oz	15	4.5	337.5
Beef Ravioli in Sauce	7.75 oz	5	3.3	247.5

CONVENIENCE FOODS (continued)

FOOD	AMOUNT	FAT GRAMS	CALORIE PTS	CALORIES
Libbys (continued):				
Beef Stew	7.75 oz	12	3.3	247.5
Chili w/ Beans	7.75 oz	12	3.8	285
Gravy w/Turkey &Drsg	7 oz.	7	2.3	172.5
Lasagna w/meat sce	7.75 oz	5	2.7	202.5
Macaroni & Beef	7.75 oz	6	3	225
Macaroni & Cheese	7.75 oz	22	4.8	360
Pasta Spirals & Chkn	7.75 oz	3	1.5	112.5
Spaghetti & Mtballs	7.75 oz	3	2.5	187.5
Corned Beef	2.3 oz.	9	2	150
Corned Beef Hash	7.75 oz.	27	5.3	397.5
Vienna Chicken Sausage	2 oz.	10	2	150
Vienna Sausage	2 oz.	15	2	150
POTATO MIXES:				
Del Monte Au Gratin	l/2 cup	11	2.5	187.5
French's Cr Ital w/parm	l/2 cup	4	1.75	131
Real Chz Scalloped	l/2 cup	5	2	150
Spuds, Mashed	l/2 cup	7	2	150
Tangy Au Gratin	l/2 cup	6	2	150
Chicken Helper	l/5 pkg	8	3.8	285
Hamburger Helper	1 cup	16	4.7	352.5
Tuna Helper	l/5 pkg	8	3.3	247.5
Inst. Potatoes (no butter)	l/2 cup	0	1.5	112.5
Lipton, Au Gratin	l/2 cup	tr	1.3	97.5
German Potato Salad	l/2 cup	tr	1.3	97.5
Italiano	l/2 cup	2	1.3	97.5
Scalloped Potatoes	7.5 oz.	16	3.5	262.5
SAUCES:				
Contadina Fr. Clam Sc	l/2 cup	15	2.5	187.5
Contadina Fr. Pesto Sc	l/2 cup	58	8	600
DiGiorino Fr. Alfredo Sc	l/2 cup	18	2.8	210
Healthy Choice Spagh	l/2 cup	0	0.5	37.5
Hunt's Spag Sc w/ Mt	l/2 cup	2	1	75
Hunts Spag Sc w/ Mush	1/2 cup	2	1	75
Newman's Spaghe Sc	l/2 cup	2	1	75
Prego Ex Chunky Sau	l/2 cup	9	2.3	172.5
Prego Spaghetti Sc	1/2 cup	6	1.8	135
Progresso Alfredo Sc	l/2 cup	30	4.5	337.5
Progresso Cr. Romano	l/2 cup	19	3	225
Progresso Wh. Clam	l/2 cup	9	1.8	135
Ragu Bf Tonight				

CONVENIENCE FOODS (continued)

FOOD	AMOUNT	FAT GRAMS	CALORIE PTS	CALORIES
Sauces (continued):				
BBQ	4 oz.	2	1	75
Lasagna	4 oz.	0	0.8	60
Stroganoff	4 oz.	0	0.7	52.5
Ragu Chickn Tonight:				
Cacciatore	4 oz.	2	1	75
Country French	4 oz.	12	1.8	135
Creamy Mush	4 oz.	10	1.5	112.5
Lt Honey Mustard	4 oz.	>1	0.7	52.5
Lt Sweet & Spicy	4 oz.	>1	0.7	52.5
Primavera	4 oz.	6	1.3	97.5
Spanish	4 oz.	2	1	75
Sweet & Sour	4 oz.	0	1	75
Ragu Garden Style	1/2 cup	2	1	75
Ragu Today's Choice	1/2 cup.	1	0.7	52.5
Wt Watchers Spaghet	1/2 cup.	2	1	75
SOUP:				
Dinty Moore Beef Stew	8 oz.	13	3	225
Hearty Soup Beef Veg	7.5 oz.	1	1	75
Hearty Chicken Noodle	7.5 oz.	3	1.5	112.5
Hormel Chili NO Bean	7.5 oz.	28	5	375
Hormel Chili w/Bean	7.5 oz.	13	3.7	281
Libby's Chili NO Bean	7.5 oz.	30	5.3	397.5
Libby's Chili w/Bean	7.5 oz.	13	3.5	263
New Eng. Clam Chowder	7.5 oz.	5	1.5	112.5

Serving Size

Is your serving the same size as the one on the label? If you eat double the serving size listed, you need to double the nutrient and calorie values. If you eat one-half the serving size shown here, cut the nutrient and calorie values in half.

Calories

Are you overweight? Cut back a little on calories! Look here to see how a serving of the food adds to your daily total. A 5' 4", 138-lb. active woman needs about 2,200 calories each day. A 5' 10", 174-lb. active man needs about 2,900. How about you?

Total Carbohydrate

When you cut down on fat, you can eat more carbohydrates. Carbohydrates are in foods like bread, potatoes, fruits and vegetables. Choose these often! They give you nutrients and energy.

Dietary Fiber

Grandmother called it "roughage," but her advice to eat more is still up-to-date! That goes for both soluble and insoluble kinds of dietary fiber. Fruits, vegetables, whole-grain foods, beans and peas are all good sources and can help reduce the risk of heart disease and cancer.

Protein

Most Americans get more protein than they need. Where there is animal protein, there is also fat and cholesterol. Eat small servings of lean meat, fish and poultry. Use skim or low-fat milk, yogurt and cheese. Try vegetable proteins like beans, grains and cereals.

Vitamins & Minerals

Your goal here is 100% of each for the day. Don't count on one food to do it all. Let a combination of foods add up to a winning score.

Nutrition Facts

Serving Size 1/2 cup (114g)
Servings Per Container 4

Amount Per Serving

Calories 90	Calories from Fat 30

	% Daily Value*
Total Fat 3g	**5%**
Saturated Fat 0g	**0%**
Cholesterol 0mg	**0%**
Sodium 300mg	**13%**
Total Carbohydrate 13g	**4%**
Dietary Fiber 3g	**12%**
Sugars 3g	
Protein 3g	

Vitamin A	80%	•	Vitamin C	60%
Calcium	4%	•	Iron	4%

* Percent Daily Values are based on a 2,000 calorie diet. Your daily values may be higher or lower depending on your calorie needs:

	Calories	2,000	2,500
Total Fat	Less than	65g	80g
Sat Fat	Less than	20g	25g
Cholesterol	Less than	300mg	300mg
Sodium	Less than	2,400mg	2,400mg
Total Carbohydrate		300g	375g
Fiber		25g	30g

Calories per gram:
Fat 9 • Carbohydrate 4 • Protein 4

More nutrients may be listed on some labels.

Total Fat

Aim low: Most people need to cut back on fat too much fat may contribute to heart disease and cancer. Try to limit your **calories from fat**. For a healthy heart, choose foods with a big difference between the total number of calories and the number of calories from fat.

Saturated Fat

A new kind of fat? No — saturated fat is part of the total fat in food. It is listed separately because it's the key player in raising blood cholesterol and your risk of heart disease. Eat less!

Cholesterol

Too much cholesterol — a second cousin to fat — can lead to heart disease. Challenge yourself to eat less than 300 mg each day.

Sodium

You call it "salt," the label calls it "sodium." Either way, it may add up to high blood pressure in some people. So, keep your sodium intake low — 2,400 to 3,000 mg or less each day.*

*The AHA. recommends no more than 3,000 mg sodium per day for healthy adults.

Daily Value

Feel like you're drowning in numbers? Let the Daily Value be your guide. Daily Values are listed for people who eat 2,000 or 2,500 calories each day. If you eat more, your personal daily value may be higher than what's listed on the label. If you eat less, your personal daily value may be lower.

For fat, saturated fat, cholesterol and sodium, choose foods with a low **% Daily Value**. For total carbohydrate, dietary fiber, vitamins and minerals, your daily value goal is to reach 100% of each.

g = grams (About 28 g = 1 ounce)
mg = milligrams (1,000 mg = 1 g)

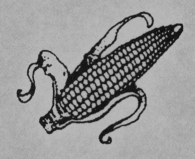

CRACKERS AND COOKIES

These snack foods may be a necessity at your house, yet serving them with fruits or vegetables or low cal beverages is wise to control portions. While many lowfat and fat free cookies are not sugar free, or low in calories, you now can find them in packs of 3-6 cookies, which is a smart buy for nibblers.

Leaving a cookie or cracker on a napkin is an excellent test for fat content. We may not notice shiny fingers, but a grease laden paper towel is obvious. Whatever you do, portion control may be the best tool to calorie and fat control. PLAN your attack, read the serving size, and then find delay techniques to stretch out snacking, and not miss the enjoyment of food that appeals to you.

Karen's Klue: Find a cracker that contains some whole grains. You will chew longer and feel full faster. Some labels will clue you into the potato chip flavor of dehydrated potatoes as an ingredient in a high fat cracker, and very little nourishment.

CRACKERS AND COOKIES

FOOD	AMOUNT	FAT GRAMS	CALORIE PTS	CALORIES
Almost Hm Choc Chip	1	3	0.8	60
Amost Hm Oatmeal R.	1	3	0.9	67.5
American Fitness Hi Energy Bar	1	2	2.8	210
Archway Bars				
Apple Bar	1	0	0.6	45
Fig Bar	1	0	0.7	52.5
Fruit Bar	1	0	1.2	90
Granola Bar	1	0	0.7	52.5
Bisco Sugar Wafers	4	3	0.9	67.5
Bisco Wafle Cremes	1	3	1	75
Bakers Bonus Oatmeal	1	3	1	75
Bloomfield Brownies	2	0	1.7	127.5
Bugs Bunny	5	2	0.8	60
Cameo Crm Sandwich	1	3	0.9	67.5
Chewy Chips Ahoy	1	3	0.8	60
CHIPS AHOY:				
Regular	1	2	0.7	52.5
Choc.Choc.Chunk	1	5	1.2	90
Reduced	3	6	2	150
Heath Toffee Chunk	1	5	1.25	94
Pecan	1	6	1.3	97.5
Rocker's Chip	1	3	0.8	60
Striped	1	5	1.3	97.5
White Fudge Chunk	1	5	1.3	97.5
COOKIES AND FUDGE:				
Grahams	1	2	0.6	45
Wafers	1	4	0.9	67.5
Striped Short Bread	1	3	0.8	60
Fat Free Apple Newton	1	0	1	75
Fat Free Fig Newton	1	0	1	75
Fig Newton	1	1	0.8	60
Fundamiddles	1 pkg	4	1.5	112.5
HEALTH VALLEY CHIPS:				
Regular	3	0	1	75
Raspberry	1	0	1.1	82.5
Strawberry	1	0	1.1	82.5
Honey Maid Cinn. Grah	2	1	0.8	60
Honey Maid Honey Gr.	2	1	0.8	60
HOMEMADE TREATS:				
Rice Krispie Treats	1 2" square	2	1	75
Toll House choc Chip	1 small	4	1.6	120

CRACKERS AND COOKIES (continued)

FOOD	AMOUNT	FAT GRAMS	CALORIE PTS	CALORIES
KEEBLER ELFIN DELIGHTS:				
Carmel Apple Oatmeal	1	1	0.7	52.5
Choc. Chip	1	2	0.8	60
Choc. Sandwich	1	2	0.8	60
Cinn Graham Crackers	8	1	0.8	60
Devils Food	1	0	1	75
Lorna Doones	2	4	1	75
Mallomar Choc. Cake	1	3	0.8	60
Mini Chips Ahoy	1	3	0.8	60
Mini Oreo Choc. Sandw	5	3	0.9	67.5
My Goodness C.C.Raisin	1	3	1.2	90
My Goodness Oat Raisin	1	3	1.2	90
Mystic Mint Sandwich	1	4	1.2	90
NABISCO:				
Chocolate Grahams	2	3	0.5	37.5
Devils Food Cake	1	1	0.9	67.5
Grahams	2	1	0.8	60
Family Choc. Wafers	2.5	2	0.9	67.5
Hey Day Bars	1	6	1.5	112.5
Ideal Bars	1	5	1.25	94
Marsh Puffs Fudge	1	4	1.2	90
Marshmallow Twirls	1	5	1.75	131
Old Fash Ginger Snaps	2	1	0.8	60
Pinweels	1	5	1.7	127.5
Pure Choc. Middle	1	5	1.1	82.5
Nilla Wafers	3.5	2	0.8	60
Nutter Butter Bite	4.5	3	1	75
Nutter Butter Sandwich	1	3	0.9	67.5
Oreo Big Stuff Ch. Sand	1	9	2.7	202.5
Oreo Choc. Sandwich	1	2	0.8	
Oreo Double Stuff Choc	1	4	0.9	67.5
Oreo Fudge Covered	1	6	1.5	112.5
PEPPERIDGE FARM GOLD FISH COOKIES:				
Chocolate	1 oz	5	1.5	112.5
Cinnamon	1 oz.	7	1.8	135
Graham	1 oz.	7	2	150
SNACKWELLS:				
Choc. Chip	6	1	0.8	60
Devils Food	1	0	0.7	52.5
Double Fudge	1	0	0.7	52.5
Oatmeal Raisin	1	1	0.8	60
Social Tea Biscuits	1	2	0.9	67.5

CRACKERS AND COOKIES (continued)

FOOD	AMOUNT	FAT GRAMS	CALORIE PTS	CALORIES
Snackwells (continued):				
Sprinkled Ch. Ahoy	1	3	0.8	60
Strawberry Newtons	1	2	0.9	67.5
SUNSHINE:				
Chips A Roos	2	7	1.7	127.5
Hydrox	3	7	2	150
Oatmeal	2	5	1.5	112.5
Strawberry Wafer ff	8	0	1.3	97.5
Sugar	2	5	1.7	127.5
Vanilla Wafers	7	6	2	150
TEDDY GRAHAMS:				
Bear/Chocolate	4	3	0.9	67.5
Bear/Cinnamon	11	3	0.9	67.5
Honey Graham	11	2	0.8	60
Vanilla Graham	11	2	0.8	60
Bearwich, Choc.& P.B.	4	3	1	75
Bearwich, Cinn & Van	4	3	1	75
Bearwich, Choc & Van	4	3	1	75
Bearwich, Grm & Choc	4	3	1	75
CRACKERS:				
Am.Cl. Cracked Wheat	4	4	0.9	67.5
Bacon Flav. Thin	7	4	0.9	67.5
Better Cheddars	10	4	0.9	67.5
Cheddar Wedges	31	3	0.9	67.5
Cheese Ritz Bits	22	4	0.9	67.5
Cheese Tid Bits	15	4	0.9	67.5
Chicken in a Biskit	7	5	1.1	82.5
Crown Pilot	1	2	0.9	67.5
Dairy Butter	4	3	0.9	67.5
Escort	3	4	0.9	67.5
FF Mister Salty Sticks	1 oz.	0	1.3	97.5
FF Prem. Crackers	5	0	0.66	49.5
FF Prem. Saltines	5	0	0.7	52.5
FF Zesta Saltines	5	0	0.7	52.5
Frookies FF	4	0	0.5	37.5
Garden Crisps	7	2	0.8	60
Harvest Crisps, 5 Grain	6	2	0.8	60
Harvest Crisps, Oat	6	2	0.8	60
Health Valley FF Crax	1/2 oz.	0	0.5	37.5
Keebler Cinnamon Cr	9	1.5	1.6	120
Keebler Honey	9	1.5	1.6	120
Keebler Wheatable	11	3	1	75

CRACKERS AND COOKIES (continued)

FOOD	AMOUNT	FAT GRAMS	CALORIE PTS	CALORIES
CRACKERS (continued):				
Low Salt Wheat Thin	8	3	0.9	67.5
Minced Onion	4	3	0.9	67.5
Mr. Phipps Pretzels	8	1	0.8	60
Mr. Phipps Pretzels Orig	1 oz.	1	1.4	105
Mr. Phipps Cheese	1 oz.	2.5	1.6	120
Mister Salty Sticks	1 oz.	1	1.5	112.5
Mister Salty Twists	1 oz.	1	1.5	112.5
Nabisco Reduce Fat:				
Better Cheddars	24	6	1.9	142.5
Town House	5	2	1	75
Triscuit	7	3	1.6	120
Wheatables	29	3.5	1.7	127.5
Wheat Thins	18	4	1.7	127.5
Nab. Ch P.B. Sandwich	4	7	1.8	135
Nab P.B.Toast	4	7	1.8	135
Old London Melba Rd	5	2	0.8	60
Old London Melba Tst	3	1	0.7	52.5
Oysterettes	18	1	0.8	60
Premium Saltine	5	2	0.8	60
Premium Soup & Oyster	20	1	0.8	60
Premium Bits	16	3	0.8	60
Premium Plus Wh Wheat	5	2	0.8	60
Ritz	4	4	0.9	67.5
Ritz Bits	22	4	0.9	67.5
Ritz Bits Cheese Sand	5	5	1.1	82.5
Ritz Bits Nacho Cheese	6	5	1.1	82.5
Ritz Bits P.B. Sand	6	4	1	75
Ryvita Crisp Bread	1	0	0.7	52.5
SNACKWELLS:				
Cheese Crackers	18	1	0.8	60
Classic Golden	6	1	0.8	60
Cracked Pepper	7	0	0.8	60
Graham Crackers	9	0	0.7	52.5
Wheat Crackers	5	0	0.66	49.5
Snorkels Cheddar	27	2	0.8	60
Snorkels Pizza	27	2	0.8	60
Sociables	6	3	0.9	67.5
SUNSHINE CRACKERS:				
Cafe	2	2	0.5	37.5
Cheezits	12	4	0.5	37.5

CRACKERS AND COOKIES (continued)

FOOD	AMOUNT	FAT GRAMS	CALORIE PTS	CALORIES
Sunshine Crackers (continued):				
Hi Ho	4	5	1	75
Honey Grahams	4	2	0.8	60
Krispy	5	1	0.8	60
Large Oyster	16	2	0.8	60
Wheat Wafers	8	4	1	75
Swiss Cheese	7	3	0.9	67.5
Triscuit Bits Wafers	15	2	0.8	60
Triscuit Wafers	3	2	0.8	60
Twiggs Sesame Cheese	5	4	0.9	67.5
Vegetable Thin	6	4	1	75
Waverly	4	3	0.9	67.5
Wheat Thins	8	3	0.9	67.5
Wheat Thins Multi Grain	8	2	0.8	60
Wheat Thins, Nutty	7	4	1	75
Wheatsworth	4	3	0.9	67.5
Cheddar Zings	15	3	1	75
Original Zings	15	3	1	75
Ranch Zings	15	3	1	75

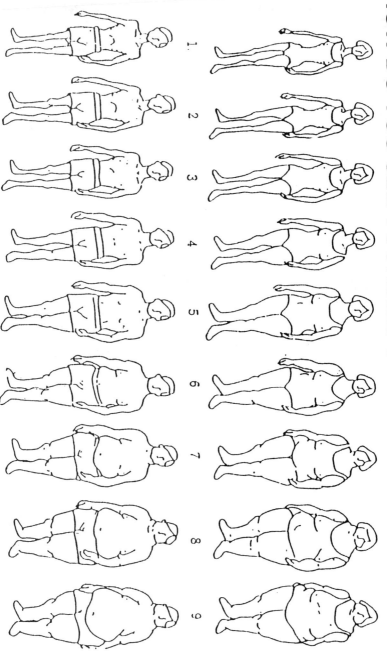

HOW DO YOU SEE YOURSELF?

48

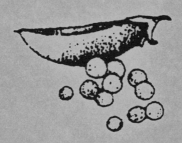

DAIRY FOODS

Milk and other dairy products are high carbohydrate foods (because cows eat grass, hay and all vegetation...) that all of us could build in higher quantities to our daily eating patterns. They are filling, come in every range of fat, and now some new "smart products" are thickened with the same culture that is in yogurt, or the whey protein that's naturally in milk for a better mouthfeel.

Because of simplesse, a fat substitute that is very safe, derived from egg whites the fat free and low fat frozen desserts that are similar to ice cream, are now creamy and very well accepted. If you haven't tasted these or yogurt for awhile, it's time. A client at a grocery store tour who had asked if she had to taste the strawberry frozen desert we were sampling, later said it was the best strawberry ice cream she had ever had (by the way of course it was her choice to taste or to not taste.)

Karen's Klue: Nestle's Quick makes a sugar free chocolate mix for cold milk that can't be beat, if you don't do well drinking it plain. Test your appetite once you've had a snack with milk and fruit, or crackers and milk, sandwich and milk...My slimmest, yet healthiest friends do!!

DAIRY FOODS

FOOD	AMOUNT	FAT GRAMS	CALORIE PTS	CALORIES
Butter	see fats			
Cream	see fats			
Margarine	see fats			
Bon Bon Ice Cream				
Nuggets, Choc.	5	12	2.3	172.5
Cocoa Bev. Mix	1 cup water	3.1	1.3	97.5
Custard	1/2 cup	7.3	2.5	187.5
Eggnog (2% milk)	1 cup	19	3	225
Ice Cream	1/2 cup	7.2	2	150
Ice Cream Bar				
(choc. coated)	1-2 oz.	10.5	2	150
Ice Cream, fat free	1/2 cup	0	1	75
ICE CREAM, NON-FAT				
MEADOW GOLD:				
Chocolate	4 oz.	0	1.2	90
Peach	4 oz.	0	1.2	90
Strawberry	4 oz.	0	1.2	90
Vanilla	4 oz.	0	1.2	90
Ice Milk, Regular	1/2 cup	5.6	1.5	112.5
Ice Milk, Soft Serve	1/2 cup	4.6	2	150
Ice Milk, Breyers Light				
Chocolate	1/2 cup	4	1.6	120
Ice Milk, Light n Lively				
Vanilla	1/2 cup	3	1.3	97.5
KRAFT NONFAT FROZEN				
DESSERT BAR:				
Chocolate Fudge	1 bar	0	1.2	90
Vanilla Fudge	1 bar	0	1	75
Vanilla Strawberry	1 bar	0	1.2	90
MILK:				
Buttermilk	1 cup	2.2	1	75
Chocolate, low fat	1 cup	5	2.5	187.5
Non-fat dried, solids	1/4 cup	0-1	1	75
Nu-Trish AB	1 cup	1	1.2	90
1% low fat	1 cup	1	1.2	90
2% low fat	1 cup	5	1.5	112.5
Skim	1 cup	0-1	1	75
Whole - 4% fat	1 cup	10	2	150
Milk Shake, Flavored	1-1/2 cup	8	5	375
Milk Shake, Malted	1-1/2 cup	9	5	375

DAIRY FOODS (continued)

FOOD	AMOUNT	FAT GRAMS	CALORIE PTS	CALORIES
PUDDINGS:				
Bread Pudding	1/4 cup	4.1	2.5	187.5
Butterscotch, Choc.				
Lemon, Tapioca,				
Vanilla	1/2 cup	4	2.5	187.5
DEL-MONTE - LITE PUDDING:				
Chocolate	4 oz.	1	1.3	97.5
Vanilla	4 oz.	1	1.2	90
Diet	1/2 cup	2	1.5	112.5
Hershey Free Pudding	1/2 cup	0	1.33	100
Jello Sugar Free made				
with skim milk	1/2 cup	0	1	75
Snack Pack				
Chocolate	4.25 oz.	7	2.2	165
Lemon	4.25 oz.	3	2	150
Vanilla	4.25 oz.	7	2.2	165
Sherbert	1/2 cup	1.9	1.5	112.5
YOGURT:				
Lowfat Plain	1 cup	3.5	1.5	112.5
Lowfat Flavored	1 cup	2.6	3	225
Blue Bunny Lite 85	8 oz.	0	1	75
Kraft Light n Lively,				
frozen, most flavors	8 oz.	0	1.2-1.4	90
TCBY, fruit flavors	5 oz. cup	0.4	2	150
TCBY, richer flavors	5 oz. cup	0.7	2.5	187.5
TCBY, sugar free,				
fat free	5 oz. cup	0	1	75
TCBY, fat free	5 oz. cup	0	1.5	112.5
Yogurt, frozen, lowfat	1/2 cup	1-3	1-1.5	75
Whole milk, flavored	1/2 cup	4	3.5	262.5
Whole milk, plain	1 cup	7.4	2	150
YOCREAM (AVAIL. AT PUMP & PANTRY):				
YoCream Premium				
Softserve	1 oz.	1	0.3	22.5
YoCream Nonfat Yogurt	1 oz.	0	0.2	15
Healthwise Milk	1 cup	0	1.2	90

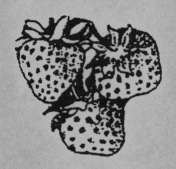

DESSERTS

If you haven't modified your old family recipes yet, you need to do so. You are naturally going to get an appetite for those foods you have fond memories of or just are in the custom of having.

Increasing fruits and grains in cookies, crisps, and any other dessert is helpful and means no flavor loss, just a real fruit flavor. Remember that sweets are a learned taste. You may have to limit baking, and buying of sweets in quantity, and instead enjoy a cone, a donut, or other sweets occasionally at a restaurant. Be sure to have a rule or guideline on these foods that you try out for a couple months if you are accustomed to them daily....

Karen's Klue: A famous restaurant in Chicago sells a 3-bite dessert, a small one inch square of 3 rich desserts that most of us love, mousse, cheesecake, etc. To most people's astonishment 3 bites may be just the right amount for taste without guilt, and even more without deprivation.

DESSERTS

FOOD	AMOUNT	FAT GRAMS	CALORIE PTS	CALORIES
Brownie (no icing):	2" square	8	2	150
Bloomfield Brownies	2 bars	0	1.7	127.5
Duncan Hines Chewy Fudge	1 as prep.	5	2	150
Duncan Hines Gourmet Mixes	1 as prep.	12	3.5	262.5
Greenfield Healthy Foods Brownie	1	0	1.6	120
Weight Watchers	1	4	1.3	97.5
CAKES (NO ICING):				
Angel Food 10"	1/12	0.2	2	150
Cheesecake 9"	1/9	16.3	4.5	337.5
Chocolate, yellow, white, etc.	1/12	11	3	225
Chocolate Covered Pops	1	8	2	150
Cupcake	1	6	2	150
Custard	1/2 cup	7.3	2.5	187.5
Del Monte Tropical Fruit Mix	0.9	1	1.3	97.5
Tahitian Tropics fruit bar	1 bar	2	1	75
FROZEN DESSERTS:				
Blue Bunny:				
Citrus Lites	1	0	0.2	15
Deluxe Fudge Lights	1	0	0.5	37.5
Nonfat Dairy Dessert	3 fl. oz.	0	0.6	45
Sugar Free Lites	1	7	1	75
Sugar Free Low Fat Dairy Dessert	3 fl. oz.	1	0.7	52.5
Klondike Lite Dessert Bar	1	6	1.5	112.5
Klondike Lite Sandwich	1	2	1.3	97.5
Healthy Choice:				
Chocolate	1/2 cup	2	1.7	127.5
Vanilla	1/2 cup	2	1.5	112.5
Lightime Yogurt Sandwiches	1	3	1.5	112.5
Lean Cuisine Ice Milk	4 fl. oz.	0	1.7	127.5
Light n Rite Vanilla Ice Cream	1/2 cup	3	1.2	90
Meadow Gold Fat Free	1/2 cup	1	1.2	90

DESSERTS (continued)

FOOD	AMOUNT	FAT GRAMS	CALORIE PTS	CALORIES
Frozen Desserts (continued):				
Quality Ck Lower in Fat				
Ice Cream Bars	1 bar	7	1.6	120
Really Vanilla Ice				
Cream	1/2 cup	2	1.3	97.5
Sealtest Fat-Free				
Dessert Bars				
Vanilla/Fudge Swirl	1 bar	0	1	75
Simple Pleasures:				
Chocolate	1/2 cup	1	2	150
Coffee	1/2 cup	1	1.5	112.5
Peach	1/2 cup	1	1.7	127.5
Rum Raisin	1/2 cup	1	1.5	112.5
Strawberry	1/2 cup	1	1.5	112.5
Toffee Crunch	1/2 cup	1	1.7	127.5
Sugar Free Eskimo Pie:				
Bar	1	11	1.8	135
Cone	1	12	3	225
Viva:				
Sugar Free Frozen				
Desert Bars	1	7	1.2	90
Sugar Free Assorted				
Pops	1	0	0.2	15
Sugar Free Fudge Bars	1	3	1	75
Weight Watchers:				
Apple Pie	1	5	2.7	202.5
Chocolate Mousse	1	6	2.2	165
Ice Cream Sandwich	1	3	2	150
Straw. Cheesecake	1	5	2.5	187.5
FROZEN PIES:				
Banquet:				
Apple	3.3 oz.	11	3.3	247.5
Banana	2.33 oz.	10	2.5	187.5
Chocolate	2.33 oz.	10	2.5	187.5
Coconut	2.33 oz.	11	2.5	187.5
Strawberry	2.33 oz.	9	2.2	165
Mrs. Smith's:				
Apple	1/8 pie	17	5.2	390
Apple Streusel	1/7 pie	16	5.5	412.5
Blueberry	1/8 pie	11	3.5	262.5
Cherry 9 5/8"	1/8 pie	11	4	300

DESSERTS (continued)

FOOD	AMOUNT	FAT GRAMS	CALORIE PTS	CALORIES
Fruitcake	1	7	2	150
Fruit Crisp	1/2 cup	3.8	2	150
Fruit Rollup	1	0	1	75
Gelatin, diet or unflavored	any amt.	0	0	0
Gelatin, plain	1/2 cup	0	1	75
Gelatin, with fruit	1/2 cup	0	1.5	112.5
Hostess:				
Cupcakes	1	6	2.2	165
HoHo's	1	6	1.5	112.5
Light Cupcake	1	2	1.7	127.5
Light Twinkie	1	2	1.7	127.5
Snoball	1	4	2	150
Twinkies	1	4	2	150
Ice Cream	see dairy			
Ice Cream Cone:				
Sugar Cone	1	0	0.5	37.5
Waffle Type	1	0	1	75
ICING:				
Buttercream (choc./vanilla)	1 T.	2.4	1	75
Choc. or Vanilla (water)	1 T.	2	1	75
White Boiled	1 T.	2	0.5	37.5
Little Debbies:				
Choc. Cakes	1 pkg.	16	4.2	315
Dessert Cups	1 pkg.	1	1	75
Devil Squares	1 pkg.	11	3.5	262.5
Fancy Cakes	1 pkg.	16	4.2	315
Fudge Brownies	1 pkg. 2 oz.	8	3.2	240
Nutty Bar	1 pkg. 2 oz.	20	4	300
Oatmeal Cremes	1 pkg. 2.17 oz.	12.6	4.5	337.5
Snack Cakes Choc.	1 pkg. 2.5 oz.	14	4.2	315
Snack Cakes Vanilla	1 pkg. 3 oz.	19	5	375
Swiss Cake Roll	1 pkg. 2 oz.	12	3.7	277.5

FOOD AND NUTRITION BOARD, NATIONAL ACADEMY OF SCIENCES — NATIONAL RESEARCH COUNCIL RECOMMENDED DIETARY ALLOWANCES,[a] Revised 1989

Designed for the maintenance of good nutrition of practically all healthy people in the United States

Category	Age (years) or Condition	Weight[b] (kg)	Weight[b] (lb)	Height[b] (cm)	Height[b] (in)	Protein (g)	Fat-Soluble Vitamins Vita-min A (ug RE)[c]	Vita-min D (ug)[d]	Vita-min E (mg α-TE)[e]	Vita-min K (ug)	Water-Soluble Vitamins Vita-min C (mg)	Thia-min (mg)	Ribo-flavin (mg)	Niacin (mg NE)[f]	Vita-min B₆ (mg)	Fo-late (ug)	Vitamin B₁₂ (ug)	Minerals Cal-cium (mg)	Phos-phorus (mg)	Mag-nesium (mg)	Iron (mg)	Zinc (mg)	Iodine (ug)	Sele-nium (ug)
Infants	0.0-0.5	6	13	60	24	13	375	7.5	3	5	30	0.3	0.4	5	0.3	25	0.3	400	300	40	6	5	40	10
	0.5-1.0	9	20	71	28	14	375	10	4	10	35	0.4	0.5	6	0.6	35	0.5	600	500	60	10	5	50	15
Children	1-3	13	29	90	35	16	400	10	6	15	40	0.7	0.8	9	1.0	50	0.7	800	800	80	10	10	70	20
	4-6	20	44	112	44	24	500	10	7	20	45	0.9	1.1	12	1.1	75	1.0	800	800	120	10	10	90	20
	7-10	28	62	132	52	28	700	10	7	30	45	1.0	1.2	13	1.4	100	1.4	800	800	170	10	10	120	30
Males	11-14	45	99	157	62	45	1,000	10	10	45	50	1.3	1.5	17	1.7	150	2.0	1,200	1,200	270	12	15	150	40
	15-18	66	145	176	69	59	1,000	10	10	65	60	1.5	1.8	20	2.0	200	2.0	1,200	1,200	400	12	15	150	50
	19-24	72	160	177	70	58	1,000	10	10	70	60	1.5	1.7	19	2.0	200	2.0	1,200	1,200	350	10	15	150	70
	25-50	79	174	176	70	63	1,000	5	10	80	60	1.5	1.7	19	2.0	200	2.0	800	800	350	10	15	150	70
	51+	77	170	173	68	63	1,000	5	10	80	60	1.2	1.4	15	2.0	200	2.0	800	800	350	10	15	150	70
Females	11-14	46	101	157	62	46	800	10	8	45	50	1.1	1.3	15	1.4	150	2.0	1,200	1,200	280	15	12	150	45
	15-18	55	120	163	64	44	800	10	8	55	60	1.1	1.3	15	1.5	180	2.0	1,200	1,200	300	15	12	150	50
	19-24	58	128	164	65	46	800	10	8	60	60	1.1	1.3	15	1.6	180	2.0	1,200	1,200	280	15	12	150	55
	25-50	63	138	163	64	50	800	5	8	65	60	1.1	1.3	15	1.6	180	2.0	800	800	280	15	12	150	55
	51+	65	143	160	63	50	800	5	8	65	60	1.0	1.2	13	1.6	180	2.0	800	800	280	10	12	150	55
Pregnant						60	800	10	10	65	70	1.5	1.6	17	2.2	400	2.2	1,200	1,200	320	30	15	175	65
Lactating	1st 6 months					65	1,300	10	12	65	95	1.6	1.8	20	2.1	280	2.6	1,200	1,200	355	15	19	200	75
	2nd 6 months					62	1,200	10	11	65	90	1.6	1.7	20	2.1	260	2.6	1,200	1,200	340	15	16	200	75

a The allowances, expressed as average daily intakes over time, are intended to provide for individual variations among most normal persons as they live in the United States under usual environmental stresses. Diets should be based on a variety of common foods in order to provide other nutrients for which human requirements have been less well defined. See text for detailed discussion of allowances and of nutrients not tabulated.

b Weights and heights of Reference Adults are actual medians for the U.S. population of the designated age, as reported by NHANES II. The median weights and heights of those under 19 years of age were taken from Hamill et al. (see pages 16-17). The use of these figures does not imply that the height-to-weight ratios are ideal.

c Retinol equivalents. 1 retinol equivalent = 1 ug retinol or 6 ug β-carotene. See text for calculation of vitamin A activity of diets as retinol equivalents.

d As cholecalciferol. 10 ug cholecalciferol = 400 iu of vitamin D.

e α-Tocopherol equivalents. 1 mg d-α tocopherol = 1 α-TE. See text for variation in allowances and calculation of vitamin E activity of the diet as α-tocopherol equivalents.

f 1 NE (niacin equivalent) is equal to 1 mg of niacin or 60 mg of dietary tryptophan.

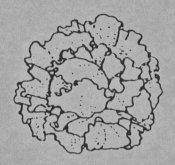

HEALTHY LIVING IN THE FAST FOOD LANE

Yes, we've all become conditioned to the fast food choices and an eating style to fit our "on the go" life styles. So the question remains how can you lower fat and calorie intake and still enjoy some foods that the chains offer.

Certainly there are high fat and highly concentrated food choices available, yet here is where your knowledge will pay off . If you have a basic idea of the fat content in a basic hamburger, fries, chicken sandwich and shake, you will be able to look at all the choices, and make a pretty good decision .You'll need to apply real meals-at least 3 food choices to your selected menu if you want to increase carbohydrates, lower fat, and most important on impulse keep you feeling fairly full. Take an apple along, a granola bar, a few crackers, and you may feel content with less fast food. Of course the great news is the choice of soups, baked potatoes, fat free dressings, and more are increasing on many fast food menus.

Remember the owners would sell more lowfat choices, if they are sure that customers will really buy a lean hamburger, and other lean choices. Supply and demand are still prevalent. Do yourself a real favor, and just as you'll read about restaurant dining, ask questions, keep sauces on the sides, and don't go in starving.

Karen's Klue: Highlight several food choices in each fast food place you frequent, for quick reference when driving up to a franchise, and in a hurry. You can save literally hundreds of calories!

FAST FOODS

FOOD	AMOUNT	FAT GRAMS	CALORIE PTS	CALORIES
AMIGOS:				
Tacos:				
Taco	1	12	2.5	188
Taco Supreme	1	14	2.84	213
Taco-Rito	1	15	4.1	308
Soft Taco	1	19	5.3	400
Chicken Soft Taco	1	11	4.4	332
Bean Tostada	1	11	3.5	259
Burritos:				
Soft Pinto	1	6	4.6	344
Crisp Pinto	1	11	3.4	252
Soft Meat	1	25	6.7	501
Crisp Meat	1	16	4.0	297
Combo	1	20	6.3	470
Veggie	1	10	4.7	355
Crisp Chicken	1	16	4.3	313
Black Bean	1	6	5.6	417
Chili	1	20	5.7	426
Cheesy	1	19	5.1	385
Salad w/o Shell/dr.:				
Sm Taco	1	15	3.0	222
Lg Taco	1	30	5.9	440
Sm Chicken Fajita	1	9	2.5	185
Lg Chicken Fajita	1	12	3.7	281
Sm Seafood	1	9	1.7	131
Sm Gr. Chicken	1	3	1.8	133
Lg Gr. Chicken	1	6	3.4	255
Black Bean	1	3	1.9	140
Chili	1	24	6.4	481
Side	1	tr	0.3	21
Sm Tortilla Bowl	1	19	3.8	287
Lg Tortilla Bowl	1	25	5.0	372
Dressings:				
Hidden Valley	2 T.	11	1.4	105
Sour Cream	2 T	4	0.7	50
Dorothy Lynch	2 T	6	1.5	110
FF Ranch	2 T	0	0.4	30
Italian	2 T	2	0.3	20
Spicy	2 T	0	0.1	8

FAST FOODS (continued)

FOOD	AMOUNT	FAT GRAMS	CALORIE PTS	CALORIES
AMIGOS (continued):				
Specialties/extras:				
Chicken Melt	1	11	3.1	230
Chicken Fajita	1	6	2.4	182
Taco Burger	1	25	6.3	474
Amigos Burrito	1	43	10.0	748
Meat Enchilada	1	40	8.9	664
Cheese Enchilada	1	32	7.3	548
Chimichanga	1	33	8.4	628
Chili	1	5	3.0	224
Chips	1	23	5.8	435
Black Beans	1	3	2.9	217
Rice	1	1	2.1	155
Refritos w/ sauce	1	5	2.9	221
ARBY'S:	1			
Roast Beef Sand.				
Arby's Melt w/ Cheddar	1	18	4.9	368
Arby-Q	1	18	5.7	431
Bac'n Cheddar Deluxe	1	34	7.2	539
Beef'n Cheddar	1	28	6.5	487
Giant Roast Beef	1	28	7.4	555
Jr. Roast Beef	1	14	4.3	324
Reg Roast Beef	1	19	5.2	388
Super Roast Beef	1	27	7.0	523
Chicken:				
Breaded Ch. Fillet	1	28	7.1	536
Ch. Cordon Bleu	1	33	8.3	623
Chicken Finger	2 pieces	16	3.9	290
Gr. Chicken BBQ	1	13	5.2	388
Grilled Chicken Deluxe	1	20	5.7	430
Roast Chicken Club	1	31	7.3	546
Roast Chicken Deluxe	1	22	5.7	433
Roast Chicken Santa Fe	1	22	5.8	436
Sub Roll Sandwiches:				
French Dip	1	22	6.3	475
Hot Ham'n Swiss	1	23	6.7	500
Italian Sub	1	36	9.0	675
Philly Beef 'n Swiss	1	47	10.1	755
Roast Beef Sub	1	42	9.3	700
Triple Cheese Melt	1	45	9.6	720
Turkey Sub	1	27	7.3	550

FAST FOODS (continued)

FOOD	AMOUNT	FAT GRAMS	CALORIE PTS	CALORIES
ARBY'S (continued):				
Light Menu:				
Rst Beef Deluxe	1	10	3.9	296
Rst Chicken Deluxe	1	6	3.7	276
Rst Turkey Deluxe	1	7	3.5	260
Garden Salad	1	0.5	0.8	61
Rst Chicken Salad	1	2	2.0	149
Side Salad	1	0.3	0.3	23
Other Sandwiches:				
Fish Fillet	1	27	7.1	529
Ham 'n Cheese	1	14	4.8	359
Ham 'n Cheese Melt	1	13	4.4	329
Potatoes:				
Cheddar Curly Fries	1	18	4.4	333
Curly Fries	1	15	4.0	300
French Fries	1	13	3.3	246
Potato Cakes	1	12	2.7	204
Bk Potato Plain	1	0.3	4.7	355
Bk Potato w/ Mar/Sr Cr	1	24	7.7	578
Broccoli'n Cheddar Pot	1	20	7.6	571
Deluxe Baked Potato	1	36	9.8	736
Soups:				
Boston Clam Chowder	1	9	2.5	190
Cr. of Broccoli	1	8	2.1	160
LumberJ. Mixed Veg	1	4	1.2	90
Old Fash. Chicken Nood	1	2	1.1	80
Potato w/Bacon	1	7	2.3	170
Timberline Chili	1	10	2.9	220
Wisconsin Cheese	1	18	3.7	280
Desserts:				
Apple Turnover	1	14	4.4	330
Cherry Turnover	1	13	4.3	320
Cheesecake Plain	1	23	4.3	320
Chocolate C. Cookie	1	6	1.7	125
Chocolate Shake	1	12	6.0	451
Jamocha Shake	1	10	5.1	384
Vanilla Shake	1	12	4.8	360
Butterfinger P.Swirl	1	18	6.1	457
Heath P. Swirl	1	22	7.2	543
Oreo P.Swirl	1	22	6.4	482

FAST FOODS (continued)

FOOD	AMOUNT	FAT GRAMS	CALORIE PTS	CALORIES
ARBYS (continued):				
Desserts (continued):				
Peanut B. C. P. Swirl	1	24	6.9	517
Snickers P.Swirl	1	19	6.8	511
Sauces & Dressing:				
Arby's Sauce	1	0.2	0.2	15
Beef Stock Au Jus	1	0	0.1	10
Bar-B-Q Sauce	1	0	0.4	30
Blue Ch. Dressing	1	31	3.9	290
Ch. Cheese Sauce	1	3	0.5	35
Honey Fr. Dressing	1	23	3.7	280
Horsey Sauce	1	5	0.8	60
Ketchup	1	0	0.2	16
Lt. Chol. Free Mayo	1	1	0.2	12
Mayonnaise	1	12	1.5	110
Mustard, German	1	0	0.1	5
Italian Sub Sauce	1	7	0.9	70
Parmesan Ch. Sauce	1	7	0.9	70
Red Ranch Dressing	1	6	1.0	75
Red. Cal Honey Mayo	1	7	0.9	70
Red Cal Ital. Dressing	1	1	0.3	20
Red Cal Butter M R.Drsg	1	0	0.7	50
Tartar Sauce	1	15	1.9	140
Thousand Isl Dressing	1	26	3.5	260
BLIMPIES:				
Sandwiches:				
Blimpies Best 6"	1	13	5.5	410
Turkey 6"	1	4.5	4.3	320
Roast Beef 6"	1	4.5	4.5	340
Cheese Trio 6"	1	23	6.8	510
Club 6"	1	13	6.0	450
Ham & Swiss 6"	1	13	5.3	400
Ham, Salami, Provolone 6"	1	28	7.9	590
Tuna	1	32	7.6	570
Gr.Chicken Salad 6"	1	12	4.7	350
Steak & Cheese	1	26	7.3	550
Gr. Chicken 6"	1	9	5.3	400
5 Meatball 6"	1	22	6.7	500
Seafood	1	20	4.0	300
Pita Pockets-Meat Ch.	1	35	4.0	300

FAST FOODS (continued)

FOOD	AMOUNT	FAT GRAMS	CALORIE PTS	CALORIES
BLIMPIES (continued):				
Dressings:				
Fat Free Ital. Dressing	1	0	0.3	20
Blue Cheese Dressing	1	24	2.9	220
Honey Fr. Dressing	1	20	3.2	240
Buttermilk Ranch	1	29	3.6	270
Thousand Island	1	21	2.8	210
Lite Italian Dressing	1	1	0.3	20
Blimpie Spec Sub	1	7	0.9	70
Lite Ranch Dressing	1	5	1.2	90
Desserts:				
Ch. Chunk Cookie	1	6.2	1.7	126
Peanut B. Cookie	1	7.5	1.8	138.3
Oatmeal Raisin Cookie	1	5	1.6	120
Condiments:				
Lettuce Topping	1	0	0.0	3.7
Tomatoes	1	0.6	0.0	3.7
Onions	1	0.3	0.1	10.9
Pita Salads of all types	1		4.0	300
BOSTON MARKET ENTREES:				
Chicken:				
1/4White Mt w/ skin	1	17	4.4	330
1/4Dk Mt No skin	1	10	0.0	210
I/4 Dk Mt w/skin	1	22	4.4	330
1/2 Chicken w/skin	1	37	8.4	630
Sknless Turkey Rot Brs	1	1	2.3	170
Original Ch. Pot Pie	1	34	10.0	750
Veg. Pot Pie	1	12	4.7	350
Chunky Ch Salad	1	30	5.2	390
Caesar	1	43	6.9	520
Caesar w/o dressing	1	13	3.2	240
Chicken Caesar Salad	1	47	8.9	670
Chicken soup	1	3	1.1	80
Ch. Brst Sandwich	1	5	5.6	420
Chunky Chi. Salad				
Sandwich	1	31	8.5	640
Turkey Sand. w/sce	1	25	8.1	610
Turkey Sandwich plain	1	2	4.8	360

FAST FOODS (continued)

FOOD	AMOUNT	FAT GRAMS	CALORIE PTS	CALORIES
BOSTON MARKET (continued):				
Steamed Vegetables	1	0.5	0.5	35
New Potatoes	1	0.3	1.9	140
Buttered Corn	1	4	2.3	190
Zucchini Marinara	1	4	1	80
Mashed Potatoes	1	8	2.4	180
Hmstyle Msh Potatoes	1	8	2.7	200
Chicken Gravy	1	1	0.2	15
Rice Pilaf	1	1	2.4	180
Cr. Spinach	1	24	4	300
Stuffing	1	12	4.1	310
Butternut Squash	1	12	2.1	160
Mac & Cheese	1	10	3.7	280
BBQ Bk Beans	1	9	4.4	330
Hot Cinn Apples	1	4.5	3.3	250
Cold Side Dishes:				
Fruit Salad	1	0.5	0.9	70
Med Pasta Salad	1	10	2.3	170
Cr.Relish	1	5	4.9	370
Cole Slaw	1	16	3.7	280
Tortellini Salad	1	24	0.5	380
Caesar Side Salad	1	17	2.8	210
Baked Goods:				
Corn Bread	1	6	2.7	200
Oatmeal R. Cookies	1	13	4.3	320
Ch. Chip Cookie	1	17	4.5	340
Brownie	1	27	6	450
BURGER KING:				
Burgers:				
Whopper	1	39	8.5	640
Whopper w/ Cheese	1	46	9.7	730
Double Whopper	1	56	11.6	870
Double Whopper w/ Cheese	1	63	12.8	960
Whopper Jr.	1	24	4.9	420
Whopper Jr. w/ Cheese	1	28	6.1	460
Hamburger	1	15	4.4	330
Cheeseburger	1	19	5.1	380
Double Cheeseburger	1	36	8	600
Double Cheeseburgerw/b	1	39	8.5	640

FAST FOODS (continued)

FOOD	AMOUNT	FAT GRAMS	CALORIE PTS	CALORIES
BURGER KING (continued):				
Sandwich/Side:				
Bk Big Fish	1	41	9.3	700
Bk Broiler	1	29	7.3	550
Chicken Sandwich	1	43	9.5	710
Chicken Tenders	6	12	3.1	230
Br. Ch. Salad	1	10	2.7	200
Garden Salad	1	5	1.3	100
Side Salad	1	3	0.8	60
French Fries (med.)	1	20	4.9	370
Onion Rings	1	14	4.1	310
Dutch Apple Pie	1	15	4.0	300
Desserts:				
Van. Shake Medium	1	6	4.0	300
Ch. Shake Medium	1	7	4.3	320
Ch. Shake Med. w/syrup	1	7	5.9	440
Strawberry Shake Med	1	6	5.6	420
Condiments:				
American Cheese	1	8	1.2	90
Mayonnaise	1	23	2.8	210
Tartar Sauce	1	19	2.4	180
Classic Blend, Low fat	1	7	0.9	65
Bulls Eye BBQ	1	0	0.3	20
Bacon bits	1	1	0.2	15
Croutons	1	1	0.4	30
Salad Dressings:				
Thous. Island Dressing	1	12	1.9	140
French Dressing	1	10	1.9	140
Ranch Dressing	1	19	2.4	180
Bleu Cheese Dressing	1	16	2.1	160
Red.Cal Ital Dressing	1	0.5	0.2	15
Dipping Sauces:				
A.M. Express Dip	1	0	1.1	80
Honey Dip	1	0	1.2	90
Ranch Dip	1	17	2.3	170
Bar B Q Dip	1	0	0.5	35
Sw & Sour Dipping Sauce	1	0	0.6	45
Breakfast:				
Croisnwhchw/ Sa,E,Ch	1	46	8.0	600
Biscuit w/Sausage	1	40	7.9	590

FAST FOODS (continued)

FOOD	AMOUNT	FAT GRAMS	CALORIE PTS	CALORIES
BURGER KING (continued):				
Breakfast (continued):				
Biscuit w/ Bacon Egg	1	31	6.8	510
French Toast Sticks	1	27	6.7	500
Hashbrown	1	12	2.9	220
A.M. Express Grape Jam	1	0	0.4	30
A.M. Express Strw Jam	1	0	0.4	30
DAIRY QUEEN BRZR:				
Small Fries	1	10	2.8	210
Large Fries	1	18	5.2	390
Soft Serve:				
Small Van. Cone	1	4	1.9	140
Large Van. Cone	1	10	4.5	340
Large Choc.Cone	1	11	4.7	350
Reg Vanilla Malt	1	14	8.1	610
Hot Fudge Br. Delight	1	29	9.5	710
Nutty Dble Fudge	1	22	7.7	580
Sm.Strb.Blizard	1	12	5.3	400
Sm. Heath Blizard	1	23	7.5	560
DQ Frozen Cake Slice	1	18	5.1	380
Reg Mr. Misty	1	0	3.3	250
Large Yogurt Cone	1	<1	3.5	260
Large Yogurt Cup	1	<1	3.1	230
Reg Strb Yog. Sundae	1	<1	2.7	200
Strb. Blizzard, Small	1	<1	3.9	290
Heath Blizzard, Small	1	12	6.0	450
QC Van.Big Scoop	1	14	4.0	300
QC Chocolate Big Scoop	1	14	4.1	310
DENNY'S FITFARE ITEMS:				
Breakfast Items:				
Buttrmlk.panw/syr.but	1 order	13	8.4	630
Pancakes	3	6	5.4	405
Syrup	2 oz.	0	2.1	157.5
Whipped Butter	1 T.	7	0.8	60
Applesauce	1serving	0	0.5	37.5
Bagel	2	1	3	225
Banana	1	1	1.4	105
Bana./strawb.medley	1 order	1	2.2	165

FAST FOODS (continued)

FOOD	AMOUNT	FAT GRAMS	CALORIE PTS	CALORIES
DENNY'S - FIT FARE ITEMS (continued):				
Breakfast Items (continued):				
Butter	1 tsp.	4	0.4	30
Cantaloupe	1/4	0	1.3	97.5
Cream of Wheat	4 oz.	1	0.8	60
Grapefruit	1/2	0	0.5	37.5
Grapes	3 oz.	0	0.7	52.5
English Muffins	1	1	2	150
Honeydew	1/4	0	1.6	120
Milk for Cereal	5 oz.	5	1.2	90
Oatmeal	4 oz.	1	0.9	67.5
Orange Juice	10 oz.	0	1.7	127.5
Salads:				
Garden Salad				
w/reduced cal. Italian	1	6	1.9	142.5
Garden Salad	1	4	1.5	112.5
Reduced cal.Italian dre	1	2	0.4	30
CA grilled chicken salad				
w/reduced cal. Italian	1	14	4.2	315
CA grilled chicken salad	1	12	3.8	285
Soups:				
Chicken Noodle Soup	1	1	0.6	45
Cream of Potato Soup	1	9	2.3	172.5
Veg. Beef Soup	1	1	0.8	60
Grilledbreast of chicken				
(with fruit-no bread)	1 order	5	2.5	187.5
Spaghetti (10 oz.) w/6oz.				
tomato (fruit-no bread)	1 order	8	8	600
Senior GrilledChicken				
w/fruit-no bread	1 order	3	1.6	120
California Blend	1 order	2	0.5	37.5
Carrots	1 order	3	1.4	105
Corn	1 order	1	1.2	90
Baked Potato	1 order	1	1.5	112.5
Green Beans	1 order	0	0.4	30
Mashed Potatoes	1 order	<1	1.1	82.5
Peas	1 order	2	1.1	82.5
Rice Pilaf	1 order	2	1.2	90

FAST FOODS (continued)

FOOD	AMOUNT	FAT GRAMS	CALORIE PTS	CALORIES
DOMINO'S PIZZA:				
Pepperoni	2 sl.	17.5	6	450
GODFATHER'S PIZZA:				
Original Crust:				
Cheese Pizza	mini/1 slice	4	1.8	135
	med/1 slice	7	3.2	240
Combo Pizza	mini/1 slice	5	2.1	157.5
	med/1 slice	12	4.2	315
Golden Crust:				
Cheese Pizza	med/1 slice	9	3	225
Combo Pizza	med/1 slice	13	3.7	277.5
GRANDMOTHERS:				
Hearty Chicken Polynes	1 serving	12.7	9.7	727.5
Hearty Chicken Sand.	1 serving	15.7	8.3	622.5
Hearty Grl Chicken Sal	1 serving	13	7	525
Hearty Halibut Steak	1 serving	15.7	9.7	727.5
Hearty Sirloin Steak	1 serving	17.3	11.8	885
HARDEE'S:				
Breakfast:				
Bacon, egg & cheese Bisc.	1	31	7	525
Bacon & egg biscuit	1	27	6.5	487.5
Bigcountrybrkfst. bacon	1	43	9.8	735
Bigcountrybrkfst.sausag	1	61	12.4	930
Biscuit N'Gravy	1	28	6.8	510
Blueberry Muffin	1	17	5.3	397.5
CanadianRiseNShineBis	1	32	7.6	570
Chicken Fillet Biscuit	1	25	6.8	510
Cinn.N'RaisinBiscuit	1	18	4.9	367.5
Country Ham Biscuit	1	22	5.7	427.5
Frisco Breakfast Sand.	1	22	6.1	457.5
Ham Biscuit	1	20	5.3	397.5
Ham,egg,& cheese bisc.	1	27	6.6	495
Orange Juice	1	0	1.8	135
Reg. Hash Brown	1	14	3	225
Rise N' Shine Biscuit	1	21	5.2	390
Sausage Biscuit	1	31	6.8	510
Sausage & Egg Biscuit	1	35	7.4	555

FAST FOODS (continued)

FOOD	AMOUNT	FAT GRAMS	CALORIE PTS	CALORIES
HARDEE'S (continued):				
Breakfast (continued):				
Steak Biscuit	1	32	7.7	577.5
Three Pancakes	1	2	3.7	277.5
3Pancakes&2baconstr.	1	9	4.6	345
3Pancakes&1saus.patt	1	16	5.7	427.5
Sandwiches:				
Bacon Cheeseburger	1	36	8	600
Big Deluxe Burger	1	30	7	525
Big Roast Beef	1	16	4.9	367.5
Cheeseburger	1	13	4	300
Chicken Fillet	1	14	5.3	397.5
Fisherman's Fillet	1	22	6.6	495
Frisco Burger	1	50	10.1	757.5
Frisco Grilled Chicken	1	34	8.2	615
Hamburger	1	9	3.4	255
Hot Dog	1	20	6	450
Hot Ham N' Cheese	1	30	7	525
MushroomN'SwissBurg.	1	27	6.9	517.5
Reg. Roast Beef	1	11	3.6	270
Quarter-Pound Ch.Burg.	1	25	6.5	487.5
Ultimate Rst. Beef Sand.	1	63	13.4	1005
Fried Chicken:				
Breasts	1	15	4.9	367.5
Leg	1	7	2.2	165
Thigh	1	15	4.4	330
Wing	1	8	2.6	195
Sides:				
Cole Slaw (4 oz.)	1	20	3.2	240
Gravy (1.5)	1	0	0.2	15
Mashed Potatoes(4 oz.)	1	0	1	75
Salads/Fries:				
Garden Salad	1	14	2.5	187.5
Chef Salad	1	13	2.5	187.5
Grilled Chicken Salad	1	4	1.6	120
Side Salad	1	0	0.2	15
Crispy Curls	1	16	4	300
French Fries(small)	1 order	10	3.4	255
French Fries(medium)	1 order	15	4.6	345
French Fries(large)	1 order	18	5.7	427.5

FAST FOODS (continued)

FOOD	AMOUNT	FAT GRAMS	CALORIE PTS	CALORIES
HARDEE'S (continued):				
Desserts:				
Big Cookie	1	12	3.7	277.5
CT Cone-chocolate	1	4	2.4	180
CT Cone-vanilla	1	4	2.4	180
CT cone-choc/van.	1	4	2.2	165
CT Sundae-Hot Fudge	1	10	4.2	315
CT Sundae-Strawberry	1	6	4.2	315
Shakes:				
Chocolate	1	10	5.2	390
Peach	1	11	7	525
Strawberry	1	8	5.2	390
Vanilla	1	9	4.9	367.5
KFC:				
KFC Original Recipe:				
Wing	1	11.75	2.3	175
Side Breast	1	16.5	3.6	274.5
Center Breast	1	15.3	3.7	281
Drumstick	1	8.5	2	150
Thigh	1	19.75	4	300
Extra Crispy:				
Wing	1	18.5	3.3	250
Side Breast	1	22.3	4.6	349.5
Center Breast	1	20	4.6	349.5
Drumstick	1	14	2.6	199.5
Thigh	1	30	5.3	400
Kentucky Nuggets	6	17.5	3	225
Nuggets Sauce all vari.	1	1	0.5	37.5
Buttermilk Biscuit	1	10	2.2	169
Mashed Potatoes w/gravy (small)	1	1.75	1	75
French Fries (small)	1	12	2.25	169
Corn on the Cob	1	3	2.3	175
Coleslaw (small)	1	6.5	1.5	112.5
Baked Beans (small)	1	2	1.75	131
Colonel Chicken Sand.	1	27.5	6.5	487.5
Rotisserie Gold Chicken:				
White Qtr. (w/skin)	6.2 oz.	18.7	4.5	337.5
Dark Qtr. (w/skin)	5.1 oz.	23.7	4.5	337.5
White Qtr. (w.o./skin)	4.1 oz.	5.9	2.6	199.5
Dark Qtr. (w.o./skin)	4.1 oz.	12.2	2.9	217.5

FAST FOODS (continued)

FOOD	AMOUNT	FAT GRAMS	CALORIE PTS	CALORIES
KFC (continued):				
Tender Roast:				
Wing w/skin	1	7.7	1.6	121
Breast w/skin	1	10.8	3.3	251
Breast w/o skin	1	4.3	2.2	169
Thigh w/skin	1	12.0	2.8	207
Thigh w/o skin	1	5.5	1/4	106
Drumstick w/skin	1	4.3	1.3	97
Drumstick w/o skin	1	2.4	.9	67
LITTLE CAESAR'S				
Baby Pan Pan	1	24.2	8.2	616
Slice, Slice	1	33.5	10.6	795
Crazy Bread	1	3.4	1.4	106
Crazy Sauce	1	0.4	1/0	74
LC Spaghetti, Little Bucket	1	12.3	7.0	528
Lasagna	1	36.6	9.6	722
Veal Parmesan	1	23.4	6.7	506
LC Spaghetti	1	6.1	3.5	264
Chocolate Ravioli Sand.	1	8.8	1.9	143
Ham & Cheese Sandwich	1	6.6	0.5	36.9
Italian Sandiwch	1	43	9.6	723
Tuna Sandwich	1	38.1	9.8	734
Vegetarian Sandwich	1	53.5	11.5	863
Big Meal Deal	1	35.9	7.1	533
Chicken Sandwich	1	24.9	7.1	531
Antipasto Salad	1	11.8	2.3	176
Caesar Salad	1	5.4	1.9	140
Tossed Salad	1	3	1.5	116
Greek Salad	1	9.6	2.2	168
Sm. Rd. Cheese Piz. Sl	1/6	6.6	2.6	193
Med. Rd. Cheese Piz. Sl	1/8	7	2.7	201
Lg. Rd. Cheese Piz. Sl	1/10	7.7	2.8	212
Sm. Rd. Cheese Piz. Pan	1/6	6.5	2.5	186
Med. Rd. Cheese Piz. Pan	1/9	6.1	2.4	181
Lg. Rd. Cheese Piz. Pan	1/12	6.5	2.5	186
Sm. Rd. Pepperoni	1/6	8.4	2.8	212
Med. Rd. Pepperoni	1/8	8.6	2.9	220
Lg. Rd. Pepperoni	1/10	9.6	3.1	233
Sm. Pepperoni Pan Pan	1/6	8.1	2.7	204
Med. Pepperoni Pan Pan	1/9	7.7	2.7	100
Lg. Pepperoni Pan Pan	1/12	8.1	2.7	204

FAST FOODS (continued)

FOOD	AMOUNT	FAT GRAMS	CALORIE PTS	CALORIES
LONG JOHN SILVERS:				
Baked Fish Dinner	1	9.5	6.9	518
Baked Chicken Dinner	1	7.5	6.0	448
Baked Combo	1	10	7.2	538
1 piece Fish	1	11	2.4	180
1 piece Chicken	1	6	1.6	120
Fish & More	1	48	11.9	890
Fish & Fry	1	37	8.1	610
3 pcs. Chicken Dinner	1	44	11.9	890
10 pcs. Shrimp Dinner	1	47	11.2	840
MCDONALD'S:				
Sandwiches:				
McRib	1	25	6.4	480
Hamburger	1	10	3.6	270
Cheeseburger	1	14	4.3	320
Quarter Pounder	1	21	5.6	420
Quarter Pounder w/cheese	1	30	7.1	530
Arch Deluxe	1	31	7.6	570
Big Mac	1	28	7.1	530
Filet-O-Fish	1	16	4.8	360
McGrilled Ckn. Classic	1	4	3.5	260
McChicken Sandwich	1	30	6.8	510
French Fries - small	1	10	2.8	210
French Fries - large	1	22	6.0	450
French Fries - super size	1	26	7.2	540
Chicken McNuggets:				
4 piece	1	12	2.7	200
6 piece	1	18	4.0	300
9 piece	1	27	6.0	450
Sauces:				
Hot Mustard	1	3.5	0.8	60
Barbecue	1	0	0.6	45
Sweet 'N Sour	1	0	0.7	50
Honey	1	0	0.6	45
Honey Mustard	1	4.5	0.7	50

FAST FOODS (continued)

FOOD	AMOUNT	FAT GRAMS	CALORIE PTS	CALORIES
MCDONALD'S (continued):				
Salads:				
Chef Salad	1	11	2.8	210
Fajita Chicken Salad	1	6	2.1	160
Garden Salad	1	4	1.1	80
Side Salad	1	2	0.6	45
Croutons	1 pkg.	1.5	0.7	50
Bacon Bits	1 pkg.	1	0.2	15
Salad Dressings:				
Blue Cheese	1 pkg.	17	2.5	190
Ranch	1 pkg.	21	3.1	230
1000 Island	1 pkg.	13	2.5	190
Lite Vinaigrette	1 pkg.	2	0.7	50
Red French Reduced	1 pkg.	8	2.1	160
Breakfast:				
Egg McMuffin	1	13	3.9	290
Sausage McMuffin	1	23	4.8	360
Sausage McMuffin/Egg	1	29	5.9	440
English Muffin	1	2	1.9	140
Sausage Biscuit	1	29	5.7	430
Sausage Biscuit/Egg	1	35	6.9	520
Bacon, Egg & Cheese Biscuit	1	27	6.0	450
Biscuit	1	13	3.5	260
Sausage	1	16	2.3	170
Scrambled Eggs	2	12	2.3	170
Hash Browns	1	8	1.7	130
Hotcakes (plain)	1	7	4.1	310
Hotcakes/marg & syrup	1	16	7.7	580
Cereals:				
Cheerios	3/4 cup	1	0.9	70
Wheaties	3/4 cup	0.5	1.1	80
Fat Free Apple Bran Muffin	1	0	2.3	170
Breakfast Danish:				
Apple	1	16	4.8	360
Cheese	1	22	5.5	410
Cinnamon Raisin	1	22	5.7	430
Raspberry	1	16	5.3	400
Cone (vanilla)	1	0.5	1.6	120

FAST FOODS (continued)

FOOD	AMOUNT	FAT GRAMS	CALORIE PTS	CALORIES
MCDONALDS (continued):				
Sundae (hot caramel)	1	3	4.1	310
Sundae (hot fudge)	1	5	3.9	290
Nuts (Sundaes)	1	3.5	0.5	40
Baked Apple Pie	1	13	3.5	260
McDonaldland Cookies	1 pkg.	9	3.5	260
Shakes (small)	1	5	4.5	340
1% Lowfat Milk (8 oz.)	1 crtn.	2.5	1.3	100
Orange Juice (6 oz.)	1	0	1.1	80
Apple Juice (6 oz.)	1	0	1.1	80
PIZZA HUT:				
(based on 1 slice of medium)				
Cheese:				
Thin 'N Crispy	1	10	3.0	223
Hand Tossed	1	9	3.4	253
Pan	1	13	3.7	279
Beef:				
Thin 'N Crispy	1	11	3.1	231
Hand Tossed	1	10	3.5	261
Pan	1	18	3.8	288
Pepperoni:				
Thin 'N Crispy	1	11	3.1	230
Hand Tossed	1	10	3.4	253
Pan	1	18	3.7	280
Italian Sausage:				
Thin 'N Crispy	1	17	3.8	282
Hand Tossed	1	15	4.2	313
Pan	1	24	5.3	399
Pork:				
Thin 'N Crispy	1	12	3.2	240
Hand Tossed	1	11	3.6	270
Pan	1	19	3.9	296
Meat Lovers:				
Thin N' Crispy	1	16	4.0	297
Hand Tossed	1	15	4.3	321
Pan	1	23	4.6	347
Veggie Lovers:				
Thin 'N Crispy	1	8	2.6	192

FAST FOODS (continued)

FOOD	AMOUNT	FAT GRAMS	CALORIE PTS	CALORIES
PIZZA HUT (continued):				
Hand Tossed	1	7	3.0	222
Pan	1	15	3.3	249
Pepperoni Lovers:				
Thin 'N Crispy	1	19	4.3	320
Hand Tossed	1	16	4.5	335
Pan	1	25	4.8	362
Supreme:				
Thin 'N Crispy	1	14	3.5	262
Hand Tossed	1	12	3.9	289
Pan	1	16	4.2	315
Super Supreme:				
Thin 'N Crispy	1	12	3.4	253
Hand Tossed	1	10	3.7	276
Pan	1	19	4.0	302
Bigfoot:				
Thin 'N Crispy	1	5	2.4	179
Hand Tossed	1	7	2.6	195
Pan	1	9	2.8	213
Chunky Meat:				
Thin 'N Crispy	1	17	3.9	295
Hand Tossed	1	16	4.3	325
Pan	1	20	4.7	352
Chunky Veggie:				
Thin 'N Crispy	1	8	2.6	193
Hand Tossed	1	6	3.0	224
Pan	1	10	3.3	251
Chunky Combo:				
Thin N' Crispy	1	12.7	3.3	250
Hand Tossed	1	11.6	3.7	280
Pan	1	13.8	4.1	306
Personal Pan Pizza:				
Pepperoni	1	29	9.0	675
Supreme	1	28	8.6	647
RUNZA:				
Runza Sandwich	1	15.31	7.2	542
Italian Runza Sandwich	1	20.21	7.0	522
BBQ Chicken Sand.	1	13.13	5.5	414

FAST FOODS (continued)

FOOD	AMOUNT	FAT GRAMS	CALORIE PTS	CALORIES
Runza (continued):				
Deluxe Chicken Sand.	1	13.11	5.4	405
Smothered Chicken	1	12.93	5.5	411
Hamburger	1	19.62	5.7	429
Deluxe Hamburger	1	26.66	6.7	506
Swiss Cheese				
Mushroom Burger	1	32.47	7.6	573
Bacon Cheese Deluxe				
Burger	1	53.44	10.9	821
Double Hamburger	1	35.55	8.8	661
Small Hamburger	1	10.79	3.6	267
Polish Dog	1	42.27	7.9	589
Fish Sandwich	1	31.9	7.9	589
Salad	1	7.35	1.4	108
Chili	1	17.55	4.4	328
Reg. Fry	1	15.86	3.4	258
Large Fry	1	22.4	4.9	365
Onion Rings	1	25.19	4.5	338
Onion Ring Dip	1	8.21	1.5	109
Brownie	1	20.89	6.2	465
Boston Clam Chowder	1	13	3.5	260
Wisconsin Cheese	1	23	4.8	360
Cauliflower Cheese	1	16	3.7	280
Vegetable Cheese	1	18.5	3.6	273
Cream of Broccoli	1	10	2.9	220
Chicken Noodle	1	2	1.6	120
Lo-Cal Italian	.5 oz.	unavail.	0.1	6
SCHOLOTZKY'S:				
Salad Dressings:				
Traditional Ranch	1	16	2.0	150
Traditional Caesar	1	20	2.5	190
Spicy Thai Peanut	1	11	1.7	130
Lemon R Vinaigrette	1	19	2.3	170
FF Ranch	1	0	0.5	40
Country French	1	15	2.5	190
Light Italian	1	3	0.5	35
Thousand Island	1	19	2.7	200

FAST FOODS (continued)

FOOD	AMOUNT	FAT GRAMS	CALORIE PTS	CALORIES
SCHOLOTZKY'S (continued):				
Salad Dressings (continued):				
Ch. Blue Cheesse	1	24	3.1	230
Honey Dijon	1	22	2.9	220
Salads:				
Greek Salad	1	13	2.6	194
Ch. Chicken Salad	1	6.1	2.5	187
Ch. Caesar Salad	1	7.5	2.3	175
Sm. Turkey Chef	1	9	3.0	223
Ch. Chef Salad	1	7.6	2.3	170
Chef Salad	1	13	3.3	248
Caesar Salad	1	2.8	0.6	45
Tossed Salad	1	1.8	0.9	65
Sandwiches:				
Original	1	33	7.8	586
Deluxe Original	1	45	10.7	806
Ham & Cheese Orig.	1	24	7.2	539
Sm. Turkey Orig	1	35	8.3	624
Sm. Turkey Breast	1	8.9	4.5	334
Ch. Breast	1	10.9	5.2	387
Dijon Ch. Breast	1	11.4	5.3	395
Vegetarian	1	10.3	4.5	334
Turkey & Bacon	1	39	8.9	668
Roast Beef & Cheese	1	29	8.2	618
Pastrami & Swiss	1	30	8.1	607
Pizza's:				
Original Combo	1	26	8.0	601
Double Ch & Pepp	1	36	9.7	727
Chicken & Pesto	1	20	8.2	616
Vegetarian Special	1	18	6.7	506
Mediterranean	1	20	7.0	527
New Orleans	1	19	8.1	606
SouthWestern	1	22	8.3	620
Double Cheese	1	20	7.1	530
Four Cheese & Tomato	1	35	9.9	745
Bar B Que Chicken	1	21.4	8.6	643
Onion & Mushroom	1	24	7.5	560
Sm. Turkey & Jalapeno	1	21	8.2	613
Bacon, Tomato & Mush	1	28	8.3	626

FAST FOODS (continued)

FOOD	AMOUNT	FAT GRAMS	CALORIE PTS	CALORIES
SUBWAY				
6" Cold Subs:				
Veggie Delite	1	3	3.0	223
Turkey Breast	1	4	3.7	276
Turkey Breast & Ham	1	4	3.7	275
Ham	1	4	3.6	273
Roast Beef	1	6	4.0	299
Subway Club	1	6	4.0	300
* Subway Seafood & Crab	1	10	4.4	333
Cold Cut Trio	1	12	4.6	347
* Tuna	1	15	5.0	372
Classic Italian B.M.T.	1	21	5.8	434
Tuna	1	33	7.0	522
6" Hot Subs:				
Roasted Chicken Breast Fillet	1	5	4.3	321
Steak & Cheese	1	10	4.8	363
Subway Melt	1	12	4.8	361
Meatball	1	15	5.5	411
Jr. Deli Style Sand:				
Turkey Breast	1	4	2.9	218
Ham	1	4	2.8	208
Roast Beef	1	5	3.1	232
* Subway Seafood & Crab	1	6	3.2	238
* Tuna	1	9	3.4	257
Subway Seafood & Crab	1	11	3.7	279
Bologna	1	11	3.6	270
Tuna	1	18	4.4	332
Jumbo Style Deli Sand:				
Turkey Breast	1	6	3.9	290
Ham	1	5	3.5	259
Roast Beef	1	9	4.5	335
* Subway Seafood & Crab	1	13	4.6	348
* Tuna	1	22	5.4	406
Bologna	1	27	5.9	446
Subway Seafood & Crab	1	27	6.3	472
Tuna	1	47	8.4	632

FAST FOODS (continued)

FOOD	AMOUNT	FAT GRAMS	CALORIE PTS	CALORIES
SUBWAY (continued):				
Salads:				
Veggie Delite	1	1	0.6	45
Turkey Breast	1	2	1.3	99
Subway Club	1	3	1.6	123
Roasted Chicken				
Breast Fillet	1	3	1.9	143
* Subway Seafood & Crab	1	8	2.1	155
* Tuna	1	13	2.6	194
Subway Seafood & Crab	1	17	3.2	238
Tuna	1	31	4.6	345
Bread Bowl	1	4	3.9	290

* Made with light mayo & no cheese or condiments.

FOOD	AMOUNT	FAT GRAMS	CALORIE PTS	CALORIES
Optional Fixin's & Condiments:				
Vinegar	1 tsp.	0	0.0	1
Mustard	2 tsp.	0	0.1	8
Light Mayo Dressing	1 tsp.	2	0.2	18
Bacon	2 slices	4	0.6	45
Cheese	2 triangles	3	0.5	41
Mayonnaise	1 tsp.	4	0.5	37
Olive Oil Blend	1 tsp.	5	0.6	45
Salad Dressings:				
Creamy Italian	1 tbsp.	6	0.9	65
Fat Free Italian	1 tbsp.	0	0.1	5
French	1 tbsp.	5	0.9	65
Fat Free French	1 tbsp.	0	0.2	15
Thousand Island	1 tbsp.	6	0.9	65
Ranch	1 tbsp.	9	1.2	87
Fat Free Ranch	1 tbsp.	0	0.2	12
Cookies:				
Oatmeal Raisin	1	6	2.0	147
Chocolate Chunk	1	7	2.1	160
Chocolate Chip	1	8	2.1	161
Toffee Crunch	1	8	2.0	153
White Chocolate Chip	1	8	2.2	166
Chocolate Chip M&M	1	8	2.2	162
Chocolate Chip Walnut	1	9	2.2	165
Peanut Butter	1	9	2.3	169
Sugar	1	9	2.4	178

FAST FOODS (continued)

FOOD	AMOUNT	FAT GRAMS	CALORIE PTS	CALORIES
SUBWAY (continued):				
Cookies:				
White Chocolate				
Macadamia Nut	1	10	2.3	174
Double Chocolate				
Brazil Nut	1	11	2.7	200
TACO BELL:				
Taco	1	11	2.4	180
Lt. Taco	1	5	1.9	140
Soft Taco	1	11	2.9	220
Lt. Soft Taco	1	5	2.5	180
Taco Supreme	1	15	3.1	230
Lt. Taco Supreme	1	5	2.7	200
Lt. Chicken Soft Taco	1	5	2.4	180
Bean Burrito	1	12	5.2	390
Lt. Bean Burrito	1	6	4.4	330
Lt. Chicken Burrito	1	6	3.9	290
Lt. 7-Layer Burrito	1	9	5.9	440
Burrito Supreme	1	19	5.9	440
Lt. Burrito Supreme	1	8	4.7	350
Taco Salad	1	55	11.5	860
Lt. Taco Salad w/ Chips	1	25	9.1	680
Lt. Taco Salad w/o Chips	1	9	4.4	330
TACO DEL SOL: (No fat content given)				
Appetizers:				
Nachos	1		10.3	771
Salsa and Chips				
Desserts:	1		5.8	436
Apple Crisp	1		3.6	272
Apple Tarta	1		4.9	369
Crispos	1		3.4	256
Salads:				
Taco Salad	1		7.2	537
Chicken Salad	1		6.6	492
Tossed Salad	1		1.0	74
Salad Dressing	1		2.9	221
Enchiladas:				
Beef	1		4.2	316
Cheese	1		5.4	406
Chicken	1		4.1	305

FAST FOODS (continued)

FOOD	AMOUNT	FAT GRAMS	CALORIE PTS	CALORIES
Taco Del Sol (continued):				
Hot Stuffed Potatoes:				
Ch & Cheddar	1		7.1	532
Sr Cream & Bacon	1		7.3	552
Potato Grande	1		10.9	820
Tacos:				
Sancho	1		5.7	431
Hardshell Taco	1		2.9	214
Softshell Taco	1		2.9	220
Specialties:				
Super Sancho	1		7.6	577
Burrito Grande	1		10.0	751
Fiesta Del Sol	1		6.3	472
Burritos:				
Combination	1		6.3	470
Beef	1		6.3	470
Bean	1		4.3	325
Tostadas:				
Combination Tostada	1		5.3	397
Beef Tostada	1		4.9	368
Bean Toastada	1		3.0	224
RefritoBeans	1		1.9	142
Taco Burger	1		4.8	361
TACO JOHN'S:				
Burritos:				
Bean Burrito	1	11	4.5	340
Beef Burrito	1	18.9	5.5	415
Combination Burrito	1	13.4	5.0	378
Super Burrito	1	18.8	5.7	424
Fajitas:				
Chkn Fajita Burrito	1	11.9	4.8	360
Chkn Fajita Salad	1	34.6	7.5	561
Chkn Fajita Softshell	1	8.3	2.9	216
Platters:				
Chimchanga	1	35.2	12.3	922
Double Enchilada	1	36.5	12.0	901
Sampler Platter	1	51	17.0	1276
Smothered Burrito Platt	1	37.5	13.0	972
Special Features:				
MexiRoll w/ Guacamole	1	46	11.2	839
Mexi Roll w/ Nacho Ch	1	43	10.8	813

FAST FOODS (continued)

FOOD	AMOUNT	FAT GRAMS	CALORIE PTS	CALORIES
TACO JOHN'S (continued):				
Mexi Roll w/ Salsa	1	37.1	10.1	754
Mexi Roll w/ Sr Cream	1	47	11.4	854
Mexican Pizza	1	36	8.5	636
Sierra Ckn Fillet Sndwh	1	21	6.7	500
Super Nachos	1	50	11.3	848
Taco Salad w/ Bowl	1	30	6.3	469
Taco's:				
Crispy Taco	1	10.3	2.4	178
Softshell Taco	1	11.3	3.7	278
Taco Bravo	1	13.6	4.4	332
Taco Burger	1	11.2	3.7	275
Side Orders/Extras:				
Beans, refried	1	7.8	4.0	301
Chili,Texas Stylew/crax	1	14.3	4.0	297
Salad Dressing,House	1	11.3	1.5	114
Mexican Rice	1	17.7	7.6	567
Nachos	1	16.8	3.9	294
Nacho Cheese	1	6	1.1	80
Potato Ole's	1	27.5	5.9	442
Potato Ole's w/ Nacho	1	33.7	7.0	523
Sour Cream	1	5.1	0.8	60
Desserts:	1			
Churro	1	7.8	2.0	147
Apple Flauta	1	1.1	1.1	84
Cherry Flauta	1	3.6	1.9	143
Cr. Cheese Flauta	1	7.9	2.4	181
Choco Taco	1	17	4.1	310
WENDY'S:				
Sandwiches:				
1/4# Hamburger Patty	1	12	2.5	190
Jr. Hamburger Patty	1	6	1.2	90
Gr. Chicken Fillet	1	2.5	1.3	100
Br. Chicken Fillet	1	10	2.9	220
Bib Bacon Classic	1	36	8.5	640
Breaded Chkn Sand.	1	25	6	450
Cheeseburger	1	13	3.6	270
Ckn Bacon Sandwich	1	26	8.1	608
Chkn Club Sandwich	1	25	6.9	518
Single w/ Everything	1	23	5.8	435
Jr. Bacon	1	25	5.8	435
Jr. Cheeseburger	1	13	4.2	315

FAST FOODS (continued)

FOOD	AMOUNT	FAT GRAMS	CALORIE PTS	CALORIES
WENDY'S (continued):				
Jr. Cheeseburger Del	1	20	5.2	390
Kaiser Bun	1	20	3	225
Sandwich Bun	1	2.5	2.1	158
Other Ingredients:	1			
Amer. Cheese	1	6	0.9	70
Amer Cheese Jr.	1	4	0.6	45
Bacon	1	2.5	0.4	30
Mayonnaise	1	7	0.9	70
Fr. Fries, Small	1	12	3.2	240
Fr. Fries, Large	1	20	5.6	420
Bk Potato, Plain	1	0	4.1	310
Bacon & Cheese	1	18	7.1	530
Broccoli & Cheese	1	14	6.1	460
Chili & Cheese	1	24	8.1	610
Sour Cr. and Chives	1	6	0.5	38
Sour Cream	1	6	0.6	42
Whipped Margarine	1	5	0.8	60
Frosty, Small	1	10	3.2	243
Frosty, Large	1	17	5.4	405
Salad Super Bar:				
Celery Seed	1	7	1.3	100
French Sw Red	1	10	1.7	130
Italian Caesar	1	16	2.0	150
Ital. Red. Fat,Red Cal	1	3	0.5	40
Salad Oil	1	14	1.7	130
Wine Vinegar	1	0	0.0	0
Garden Spot Bar:				
Applesauce	2 T.	0	0.4	30
Bacon Bits	2 T.	1.5	0.5	40
Cantaloupe Sliced	1 pc.	0	0.2	15
Carrots	1/4 cup	0	0.1	5
Cauliflower	1/4 cup	0	0.0	0
Cheddar Chips	2 T	4	0.9	70
Cheese, Shredded,Imit	2 T.	4	0.7	50
Chicken Salad	2 T.	5	0.9	70
Chives	1 T.	0	0.0	0
Chow Mein Noodles	1/4 c.	2	0.5	35
Cole Slaw	2 T.	3	0.6	45
Cottage Cheese	2 T.	1.5	0.5	40
Croutons	2 T.	1	0.4	30
Cucumber	2 sl	0	0.0	0
Eggs, Hard Cooked	2 T.	3	0.5	40

FAST FOODS (continued)

FOOD	AMOUNT	FAT GRAMS	CALORIE PTS	CALORIES
WENDY'S (continued):				
Green Peas	2 pc.	0	0.2	15
Green Peppers	2 pc.	0	0.0	0
Honeydew Melon	1 pc.	0	0.3	20
Jalapeno Pepper	1 T.	0	0.0	0
Lettuce	1 c.	0	0.1	10
Mushrooms	1/4 c.	1	0.0	0
Olives, Black	2 T.	1.5	0.2	15
Orange Section	1 pc.	0	0.1	10
Pasta Salad	2 T.	0	0.3	25
Peaches, Slices	1 slice	0	0.2	15
Pepperoni, Sliced	6 sl.	3	0.4	30
Pineapple Chunks	4 pc.	0	0.3	20
Potato Salad	2 T.	7	1.1	80
Pudding, Choc	1/4 c.	3	0.9	70
Pudding, Van	1/4 c.	3	0.9	70
Red Onions	3 rings	0	0.1	10
Seafood Salad	1/4 c.	4	0.9	70
Sesame Breadstick	1	0	0.2	15
Strawberries	1	0	0.1	10
Strawberry Banana Des	1/4 c.	0	0.4	30
Sunflower Seeds & Raisin	2 T.	5	1.1	80
Tomato Wedges	1 pc.	0	0.1	5
Turkey Ham, Diced	2 T.	4	1.2	90
Watermelon, Wedge	1 pc.	0	0.3	20

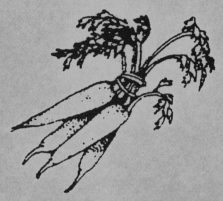

FATS

We put salad dressing and sauces under the fats listing for a good reason, your awareness of what your taking in...and of course today there are excellent products with low or no fat contained.

Creaminess is a favorite texture in many dishes, and you may want to modify the sauce first with part regular, and part fat free product to test for taste, and consistency. The stores have new products constantly yet, in the Midwest and smaller populations new products often come and go before we have a chance to test them out, and vote our approval.

Karen's Klue: Fat free sour cream in dips, and baked products is excellent. Use it to replace much of the fat, and in quick breads, and muffins you may have a moister and higher quality product than even before.......

FATS

ITEM	AMOUNT	FAT GRAMS	CALORIE PTS	CALORIES
Au jus	1/2 cup	0	0.2	19
Butter	1 tsp.	5	0.5	37.5
Cheese Sauce	1/4 cup	4.1	2	150
Cocktail Sauce	1/4 cup	0	1	75
Coffee Mate Light	1 T.	1	.1	10
Creams:				
Half & Half	1 T.	3	0.2	19
Imitation Sour Cream	3 T.	6.9	1	75
Liquid	2 T.	3	0.5	37.5
Lite Sour Cream	3 T.	3	0.5	37.5
Non-dairy Creamer	3 1/2 tsp.	2.5	0.5	37.5
Non-dairy Whipped Topping	3 T.	2	0.5	37.5
Non-fat Sour Cream, Daisy	2 T.	0	0.3	19.5
Reduced Cal. Non-Dairy Creamer	3 1/2 tsp.	1.5	0.5	37.5
Sour Cream	3 T.	7.5	1	75
Whipped Cream	3 T.	2.1	2	150
Whipped Topping Mix	2 T.	1	0.5	37.5
Whipped Topping Mix, diet	2 T.	1.2	0	0
Dressings:				
Blue Cheese, Roquefort	2 T.	8.6	2	150
Coleslaw	2 T.	5	2.5	187.5
Creamy type, Cucumber, Green Goddess, Italian, Onion,	2 T.	14	2	150
French, Russian	2 T.	13.8	1.5	112.5
Dorothy Lynch Reduced Cal	1 T.	1	0.5	37.5
Good Seasons Italian	1 T.	8	1	75
Good Seasons Italian Lite	1 T.	3	0.3	25
Good Seasons Zesty Italian	1 T.	8	1	75
Healthy Sensation Dressing:				
Chunky Blue Cheese	2 T.	0	0.5	37.5
French	2 T.	0	0.5	37.5
Honey Dijon	2 T.	0	0.6	49.5
Italian	2 T.	0	0.2	19

FATS

ITEM	AMOUNT	FAT GRAMS	CALORIE PTS	CALORIES
Healthy Sensation Dressing (continued):				
Ranch	2 T.	0	0.5	37.5
Thousand Island	2 T.	0	0.5	37.5
Hidden Valley Red.				
Calorie Homemade	1 T.	3	0.5	37.5
Italian Oil & Vinegar	2 T.	14.2	2	150
Kraft Catalina fat free	2 T.	0	0.5	37.5
Kraft French &				
1000 Island fat free	2 T.	0	0.5	37.5
Kraft Italian, Viva				
Italian, Red Wine				
Vinegar, fat free	2 T.	0	0.2	19
Kraft Ranch fat free	2 T.	0	0.5	37.5
Kraft Rancher's				
Choice - diet	2 T.	6	1	75
Kraft Reduced Bacon				
& Tomato, Chunky				
Blue Cheese. Creamy				
Bacon, Creamy Italian,				
House & Zesty Italian	2 T.	4	0.7	56
Kraft Reduced				
Catalina, French,				
Russian, 1000 Island	2 T.	2	0.5	37.5
Kraft Reduced				
Buttermilk	2 T.	6	1	75
Kraft Roka Cheese	2 T.	2	0.5	37.5
Ranch or Homestyle	2 T.	11.4	1.5	112.5
7 Seas Buttermilk	2 T.	10	1.3	100
7 Seas French	2 T.	6	1	75
7 Seas 1000 Island	2 T.	4	1	75
7 Seas Ranch	2 T.	10	1.3	100
7 Seas Red Wine,				
Vinegar & Oil	2 T.	8	1	75
7 Seas Viva				
Creamy Italian	2 T.	8	1.2	94
7 Seas Viva				
Herbs & Spices	2 T.	6	1	75
7 Seas Viva Italian	2 T.	6	1	75
Spin Blend				
Fat Free Dressing	1 T.	0	0.2	15
Thousand Island	2 T.	11.2	2	150

FATS

ITEM	AMOUNT	FAT GRAMS	CALORIE PTS	CALORIES
Gravy, Avg., Homemade	4T.	20	3	225
Gravy Mix	1/2 cup	3.4	0.6	49.5
Hollandaise Sauce	14 cup	3	0.5	37.5
Horseradish Sauce	2 T.	2.6	1	75
I Can't Believe It's Not Butter	1 T.	7	0.7	56
Land O Lakes No Fat Sour Cream	2 T.	0	0.5	37.5
Margarine	1 tsp.	5	0.5	37.5
Margarine, Diet	2 tsp.	2.5	0.5	37.5
Mocha Mix Light	1 T.	1	0.1	10
Oils, Vegetable, any	1 tsp.	4.5	0.5	37.5
Promise Ultra Margarine	1 T.	4	0.5	37.5
Promise Ultra Fat Free	1 T.	0	0	5
Sauces: Barbecue, Catsup, Chili	1/4 tsp.	1.2	1	75
Shortening, Vegetable	1 tsp.	4	0.5	37.5
Sour Cream/ Stroganoff Mix	1/4 cup	7.1	1.5	112.5
Soy Sauce	2 T.	0	0	0
Suet	1 T.	13.1	0.5	37.5
Sweet & Sour Sauce	2 T.	0.1	0.5	37.5
Taco Sauce	1 T.	0	0	0
Tarter Sauce	1 T.	7.9	1.5	112.5
Teriyaki Sauce	2 T.	0	0.4	30
Weight Watchers Extra Light Spread	1 T.	4	0.6	19.5
White Sauce	1/4 cup	4	1.5	112.5
Worcestershire Sauce	1 T.	0	0	0

FOOD CONTROL METHODS

#1 Use delay technique: Any time you feel like eating inappropriately, delay the decision 10-15 minutes. Do not tell yourself NO. At the end of the fifteen minute time period, you may decide you can eat, you may change the choices, and you may decide it was not necessary. With time you can increase the delay period to 30 minutes. Be strict with yourself using the clock. Controlling the behavior, and impulse for your best decision is your real goal.

#2 Ask yourself when you are wanting food, and should not be physically hungry, or have just eaten, these 3 questions:
  1-What is bothering me right now?
  2-What will food do for me?
  3-What can I do to feel better right now, other than food?

#3 Facts versus Feelings: We need to use external and internal cues to determine our need to eat. The facts will tell you when you last ate, the quantity, or fat grams, and how much physical activity planned for the day....in essence, should you really eat?

Your feelings will not give you objective information, but aid the need to feed your appetite. When you sort facts and feelings you will come to a better decision for your body!

As someone new to daily delaying, use only #1 at first. The other control methods can be used as time and you progress.

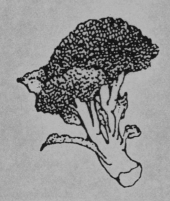

FISH, MEAT AND POULTRY

Our section on meat illustrates the importance of portion control, but also the variation in fat and calories from different cuts of meats....Most Americans eat about 200% of their protein needs, and yet are low in carbohydrates and vitamins, minerals and fiber. If you have felt meat was high fat, then you may have decreased these choices to a level where you are over-hungry, and over eat on low nutrient foods.

Six ounces a day for females, and 8 ounces average for males is a good amount to supply protein needs without excess calories or fat. Lean is truly the name of the game, and if you've been of the belief that one meat is always leaner than another.....THINK AGAIN.

FISH, MEAT AND POULTRY

ITEM	AMOUNT	FAT GRAMS	CALORIE PTS	CALORIES
FISH:				
Anchovy, raw	3 oz.	4.11	1.5	112.5
Bass, freshwater raw	3 oz.	3.18	1.3	101
Carp, raw	3 oz.	4.8	1.5	112.5
Catfish,				
Channel, raw	3 oz.	4.8	1.5	112.5
Caviar, black &				
red, granular	3 oz.	2.9	0.5	37.5
Clams, raw	3 oz.	0.8	0.8	60
Cod, Atlantic raw	3 oz.	1.2	1	75
Cod, breaded,				
Van de Kamps	3 oz.	20	3.9	292.5
Cod, Pacific, raw	3 oz.	0.5	0.9	67.5
Crab, Alaska King raw	3 oz.	0.5	0.9	67.5
Imitation, made				
from surimi	3 oz.	1.11	2.5	187.5
Fish Fillets, frozen	3 oz.	9.99	2.5	187.5
Fish Sticks, frozen	1 stick	3.4	1	75
Batter-dipped				
Van de Kamps	3 oz.	45	9	675
Fisher Boy Fish Sticks	3 sticks	5	2.2	169
Flounder/Sole	3 oz.	0.5	1	75
Haddock, raw	3 oz.	0.6	1	75
cooked by dry heat	3 oz.	0.81	1.3	97.5
Halibut, Atlantic				
& Pacific raw	3 oz.	2	1.2	90
Halibut, fz batter-dipped				
Van de Kamps	3 oz.	15	3	225
Herring, Atlantic raw	3 oz.	7.71	2	150
Pickled 1 piece	3 oz.	4.5	3.7	281
Lobster, Northern raw	3 oz.	0.81	1	75
Oysters, Pacific raw	3 oz.	2	1	75
Perch, raw	3 oz.	0.81	1	75
Pike, Walleye, raw	3 oz.	1	1	75
Pollock, Atlantic raw	3 oz.	0.81	1	75
Pollock, Walleye raw	3 oz.	0.81	1	75
Rockfish, Pacific raw	3 oz.	1.29	1	75
Roughy, Orange, raw	3 oz.	6	1.5	112.5
Salmon, chim	3 oz.	0.81	1.5	112.5
Salmon, chinook	3 oz.	8.91	2	150
Salmon, pink	3 oz.	2.91	1.3	97.5
Sardines, Atlantic,				
2 in soybean oil	3 oz.	8.4	2.2	169

FISH, MEAT AND POULTRY

ITEM	AMOUNT	FAT GRAMS	CALORIE PTS	CALORIES
FISH (continued):				
Scallops, raw	3 oz.	1.5	1.2	94.5
Shrimp, raw	3 oz.	1.5	1.2	94.5
breaded & fried	11 large	30.3	8.2	619
Snapper, raw	3 oz.	1.1	1.2	94.5
Sole	3 oz.	0.5	1	75
Squid	3 oz.	1.4	0.75	56
Trout, Rainbow, raw	3 oz.	2.9	1.3	97.5
TUNA: Canned in oil	3 oz.	6.9	2.3	172.5
Light, chunk	3 oz.	12.9	2.3	172.5
Canned in spring water	3 oz.	0.39	1.5	112.5
Whitefish, raw	3 oz.	5	1.5	112.5

THE SKINNY SIX

All of the following six cuts of meat are know as the skinny six. This means that they are each under 175 calories or 2.33 points or less for 3 oz. cooked meat. They also contain only 8.5 or less grams of fat for 3 oz. cooked trimmed serving.

ITEM	AMOUNT	FAT GRAMS	CALORIE PTS	CALORIES
Eye of Round	3 oz. cooked	4.2	2	150
Round Tip	3 oz. cooked	5.9	2	150
Sirloin	3 oz. cooked	6.1	2.3	172.5
Tenderloin	3 oz. cooked	8.5	2.3	172.5
Top Loin	3 oz. cooked	8	2.3	172.5
Top Round	3 oz. cooked	4.2	2	150

FISH, MEAT AND POULTRY

ITEM	AMOUNT	FAT GRAMS	CALORIE PTS	CALORIES
OTHER LOWFAT MEATS 7.5-12.4% fat cooked:				
Arm/blade lean				
pot roast	3 oz.	3	3	225
Dried Beef	3 oz.	5.4	2.2	169
Flank Steak	3 oz.	12	3	225
Healthy Choice				
Hamburger	3 oz.	7.7	2.7	200
Liver, Heart etc	3 oz.	3.6	3	225
5% Lean				
Ground Beef	3 oz.	7.7	2.7	200
Medium Fat				
Meats in general	3 oz.	15	3	225
Corned,				
Pastrami, Lean	3 oz.	12	3	225
80% Lean				
Ground Beef	3 oz.	12	3	225
Prime Rib, 1/4"				
fat trim	3 oz.	15.6	3.2	240
Stew Meat, Roast	3 oz.	15	3	225
High Fat Meats:				
Brisket Lean				
& Marbled	3 oz.	22.3	4.65	349
Rib-eye Steak	3 oz.	22.3	4.65	349
Rib Roast	3 oz.	30	5	376
Short Ribs	3 oz.	40	6	450
Sirloin, Ground	3 oz.	32	5	376
Steak, Chicken Fried	3 oz.	30	5	376
T-Bone	3 oz.	30	5	376
HOT DOGS:				
Healthy Choice				
Beef Franks, 8 ct.	1	1	0.8	60
Bunsize, 8 ct.	1	2	0.9	67.5
Jumbo, 8 ct.	1	2	0.9	67.5
Regular, 10 ct.	1	1	0.5	37.5
Hormel Light & Lean	1	1	0.7	56
Light & Mild Jumbo Franks	1 link	8	1.5	112.5
Louis Rich				
Light Hot Dogs	1	8	1.3	100
Morning Star				
Meatless Grillers	1 (2.25oz.)	7	2	150

FISH, MEAT AND POULTRY

ITEM	AMOUNT	FAT GRAMS	CALORIE PTS	CALORIES
HOTDOGS (continued):				
Oscar Mayer :				
Bun Length	1	17	2.5	187.5
Light Hot Dog	1	11	1.7	131
Wieners	1	13	2	150
BUFFALO:	3 oz.	1.98	1.5	112.5
LAMB:				
Chop, Lean Roast	3 oz.	18	9	675
HAM:				
Cured Butt, Lean	3 oz.	3.87	1.2	89
Cured Lean	3 oz.	8.58	2.8	209
Fresh Lean	3 oz.	5.49	2.6	193.5
Shoulder Lean	3 oz.	4.71	1.7	128
Smoked	3 oz.	9.42	2	151
PORK:				
Bacon, raw	3 oz.	48	6	450
Canadian Bacon	3 oz.	15	3	225
Lean Ground Pork	3 oz.	15	3	225
Pork Center				
Loin Chop	3 oz.	6.9	2.2	169
Pork Loin Roast,				
Boneless	3 oz.	6	2.2	169
Pork Top Loin				
Chop Boneless	3 oz.	6.6	2.2	169
Sirloin Chop	3 oz.	5.7	2.2	169
Spareribs, meat only	2 lg.	12	1.5	112.5
Tenderloin	3 oz.	4.11	1.8	135
SAUSAGE:				
Bulk, patties	1 oz.	7	1.5	112.5
Italian	1 link	15	4	300
Links	1/10lb.	12	2	150
Polish	1	15	4	300
Polish Sausage				
Oscar Mayer	1 (2.7 oz.)	20	3	225
Vienna, canned	2	8	1.3	97.5
Louis Rich Turkey				
Smoked Sausage	3 oz.	6	1.5	112.5
RABBIT	3 oz.	5.25	1.5	112.5
VEAL:				
Chop, Roast, Steak	3 oz.	27	3	225
Cutlet	3 oz.	33	4.5	337.5

FISH, MEAT AND POULTRY

ITEM	AMOUNT	FAT GRAMS	CALORIE PTS	CALORIES
Deli Meats:				
Deli Select	1 sl.	<1	0.25	19
Emmber Lean &				
Tender, Corned Beef,				
Pastrami, & Italian				
Beef	1 sl.	1	0.25	19
Festival Foods Deli Meats:				
Ham	1 oz.	1	0.4	30
Hard Salami	3 slices	9	1.4	105
Honey Ham	1 oz.	1	0.5	34.5
Lite Roast Beef	1 oz.	1	0.3	22.5
Turkey Breast	1 oz.	0.5	0.4	30
Healthy Choice Packaged Meats:				
Regular Sliced				
Cold Cuts (2 oz. = 2 slices)				
Baked/Cooked Ham	2 sl.	2	0.8	60
Honey Roasted				
& Smoked				
Turkey Breast	2 sl.	2	0.9	67.5
Oven Roasted				
Chicken Breast	2 sl.	1	0.8	60
Oven Roasted				
Turkey Breast	2 sl.	2	0.8	60
Smoked Chicken				
Breast	2 sl.	1	0.8	60
Smoked Ham	2 sl.	2	0.8	60
Smoked				
Turkey Breast	2 sl.	2	0.8	60
Turkey Ham	2 sl.	2	0.8	60
Regular Sliced Cold Cuts (2 oz. = 3 slices):				
Beef Bologna	3 sl.	2	0.8	60
Bologna	3 sl.	2	0.8	60
Deli Thin Sliced Cold Cuts (2 oz. = 6 slices):				
Baked/Cooked Ham	6 sl.	2	0.9	67.5
Bologna	6 sl.	2	0.8	60
Cooked Ham	6 sl.	1	0.8	60
Honey Ham	6 sl.	2	0.8	60
Honey Roasted &				
Smoked Turkey				
Breast	6 sl.	2	0.9	67.5
Oven Roasted				
Chicken Breast	6 sl.	1	0.8	60

FISH, MEAT AND POULTRY

ITEM	AMOUNT	FAT GRAMS	CALORIE PTS	CALORIES
Deli Meats (continued):				
Oven Roasted				
Turkey Breast	6 sl.	2	0.8	60
Roast Beef	6 sl.	2	0.9	67.5
Smoked Chicken				
Breast	6 sl.	1	0.8	60
Smoked Ham	6 sl.	1	0.8	60
Smoked				
Turkey Breast	6 sl.	2	0.8	60
Turkey Ham	6 sl.	2	0.8	60
Low Fat Sausage:				
Low Fat Smoked				
Sausage rope	2 oz.	2	0.9	67.5
Low Fat Polska				
Kiebasa, rope	2 oz.	2	0.9	67.5
Low Fat Ground				
Beef Product	4 oz.	4	1.7	127.5
Hillshire Farm Meats:				
Braunschwieger	1 oz.	8	1.3	100
Bun Size				
Cheddarwurst	1	18	2.6	200
Bun Size				
Smoked Sausage	1	16	2.5	187.5
Bun Size Wieners	2 oz.	16	2.3	175
Cheddar Hots				
(80% fat free)	2 oz.	12	2	150
Cheddarwurst	2 oz.	17	2.5	187.5
Fresh Bratwurst	2 oz.	17	2.5	187.5
Hot Links	1	16	2.5	187.5
Kielbasa				
(80% fat free)	2 oz.	10	1.6	124.5
Light Fresh				
Bratwurst	2 oz.	11	2	150
Lit'l Smokies	2 oz.	8	1.7	131
Light Mild & Hot				
Italian Sausage	2 oz.	11	2	150
Light Summer				
Sausage	2 oz.	12	2	150
Lite Cheddarwurst	2 oz.	15	2.5	187.5
Lite Hot Links	1	15	2.5	187.5

FISH, MEAT AND POULTRY

ITEM	AMOUNT	FAT GRAMS	CALORIE PTS	CALORIES
Hillshire Farm Meats (continued):				
Lite Polska Kielbasa				
& Smoked Sausage	2 oz.	11	1.7	131
Lit'l Beef Franks	2 oz.	16	2.3	175
Lit'l Smokies	2 oz.	16	2.5	187.5
Lit'l Wieners	2 oz.	16	2.3	175
Mild & Hot				
Italian Sausage	2 oz.	1	2	150
Ring Bologna	1 oz.	8	1.3	100
Smokies				
(80% fat free)	2 oz.	10	1.6	124.5
Summer Sausage	2 oz.	16	2.3	175
Turkey Polska				
Kielbasa	2 oz.	5	1.2	94
Turkey Smoked				
Sausage	2 oz.	5	1.2	94
VEGETABLE SOURCES OF PROTEIN:				
BAMA Jelly &				
Peanut Butter	2 T.	7	1.5	112.5
Beans, dried, cooked:				
Great Northern,				
Navy, Soybeans	1/2 cup	0	1.5	112.5
Beans, canned:				
Bush's Baked Beans	4 oz.	1	1.6	124.5
Bush's Pork & Beans	4 oz.	1	1.6	124.5
Garbonzo, Kidney,				
Lima, Red, Refried	1/2 cup	1	1.5	112.5
Lentils, cooked	1/2 cup	0	1	75
Van De Kamps				
pork & beans	6 oz.	1	2	150
Eggs (large)	1	6	1	75
Egg Substitute				
Country Morning				
Land O Lakes	1/2 cup	12.1	2.3	172.5
Egg Beaters				
Fleishchman's	1/4 cup	0	0.33	25
Scramblers,				
Morning Star	1/4 cup	2.4	0.7	52.5
Nuts Roasted:				
Almonds, Cashews,				
Peanuts, Pecans,				

FISH, MEAT AND POULTRY

ITEM	AMOUNT	FAT GRAMS	CALORIE PTS	CALORIES
Vegetable Sources of Protein (continued):				
Peanut Butter:				
Jif Creamy & Crunchy	2 T.	16	2.5	187.5
Jif Reduced Fat	2 T.	12	2.5	187.5
Peter Pan Whipped	2 1/2 T.	16	1.5	112.5
Skippy, Creamy &				
Crunchy	2 T.	17	2.5	187.5
Skippy, Reduced Fat	2 T.	12	2.5	187.5
Peas, Dried, Cooked:				
Blackeyed Peas,				
Cowpeas, Split Peas	1/2 cup	0	2	150
Tofu Firm & Raw	3 oz.	6	1.25	93.75
CHICKEN (avg. 3.5 oz.):				
Breast				
w/skin, fried	1/2 breast	11	3	225
w/o skin, fried	1/2 breast	6	2.5	187.5
w/skin, roasted	1/2 breast	7.5	2.6	199.5
w/o skin, roasted	1/2 breast	3	2	150
Fryers				
w/skin batter dipped				
& fried	1 oz.	5	1.2	94
w/skin, roasted	1 oz.	3.86	0.8	64.5
Giblets, fried	3 1/2 oz.	13.5	3.6	274.5
Leg (avg. 1.5 oz.)				
w/skin, fried	1 leg	9	1.6	124.5
w/skin, roasted	1 leg	6	1.5	112.5
w/o skin, roasted	1 leg	2.5	1	75
Stewers				
w/skin	1 oz.	5.43	1.1	80
w/o skin	1 oz.	3.43	0.64	48
Thigh (avg. 1 oz.)				
w/skin, fried	1 thigh	11	2.5	187.5
w/skin, roasted	1 thigh	6	1.5	112.5
w/o skin, roasted	1 thigh	5.5	1.5	112.5
Wing (avg. 1 oz.)				
w/skin, fried	1 wing	9	1.6	124.5
w/skin, roasted	1 wing	6.5	1.3	97.5
Chicken by George:				
Cajun Style	5 oz.	9	2.6	199.5
Caribbean Grill	5 oz.	4	2.3	175
Italian Style				
Blue Cheese	5 oz.	8	2.5	187.5

FISH, MEAT AND POULTRY

ITEM	AMOUNT	FAT GRAMS	CALORIE PTS	CALORIES
Chicken by George (continued):				
Blue Cheese	5 oz.	8	2.5	187.5
Lemon Herb	5 oz.	4	2	150
Mesquite Barbecue	5 oz.	4	2.2	169
Mexican Style	5 oz.	9	2.6	199.5
Mustard & Dill	5 oz.	7	2.3	175
Teriyaki	5 oz.	4	2.3	175
Tomato Herb w/basil	5 oz.	7	2.5	187.5
Canned Chicken:				
Swanson Chicken w/broth	1 oz.	2.4	0.6	45
Swanson Chunk Mixin	1 oz.	3.2	0.7	52.5
Swanson Chunk Premium White	1 oz.	0.8	0.4	30
TURKEY:				
Dark meat w/skin roasted	1 oz.	3.29	0.9	72
Dark meat w/o skin roasted	1 oz.	2.07	0.7	54
Light meat w/skin roasted	1 oz.	2.38	0.7	57
Light meat w/o skin roasted	1 oz.	0.93	0.6	43
Ground	1 oz.	4	0.8	37.5
Turkey Bacon	1 strip	3	0.5	37.5
Louis Rich Turkey Breast:				
Barbecue	1 oz.	1.43	0.5	37.5
Oven Roasted	1 oz.	0.86	0.4	32
Smoked	1 oz.	1.14	0.5	35
Louis Rich Turkey Breast, fat free	1 sl.	0	0.3	22.5
Deli Meats Turkey:				
Turkey Breast	1 oz.	1.5	0.5	37.5
Turkey Ham	1 oz.	1.5	0.5	37.5
Turkey Pastrami	1 oz.	1.75	0.6	49.5
Turkey Roll	1 oz.	4.5	1	75
Turkey Salami	1 oz.	3.75	0.7	56
OTHER POULTRY:				
Duck, meat only	1 oz.	3	0.7	56
Pheasant with or without skin, cooked	1 oz.	2.71	0.8	64.5
Quail with or without skin, cooked	1 oz.	2.7	0.8	64.5

HOW MUCH MEAT SHOULD YOU EAT

Knowing how much meat you are taking in is a real key to long-term success in controlling fat gram intake, weight and cholesterol. General guidelines for adult females include 4-6 oz. protein/day and for adult males 6-8 oz./day. For other age groups or special health needs contact a dietitian or physician to calculate your personal protein needs. Exercise, milk product intake, illness, weight, medication and many other factors contribute to this. Just as it may take some time to get your fat gram intake to the levels indicated earlier in the book, give yourself time to also decrease meat to these levels. You can increase complex carbohydrates low in fat content, while cutting back on meat portions and still supply nutrients and energy necessary to your optimal health.

SUGGESTIONS FOR CONTROLLING MEAT PORTIONS:

1. Measure meat whenever possible with an ounce scale.

2. A deck of cards is approximately three ounces of meat when you have to estimate.

3. Cut off any visible fat, and rinse. Drain or find any other way to remove fats in broths and juices. You will save "hundreds" of unnecessary calories for your body to digest.

4. Allow yourself a variety of meat, including red to satisfy your tastebuds, and B-vitamin and iron needs. The great dieters have lived on one or two types of lean meats for months and years, and set themselves up to "fail" and go off their plan.

5. If you're not sure of the fat content of meat ,you may use the following:
   AN OUNCE OF MED. FAT MEAT = 5 GRAMS OF FAT
   AN OUNCE OF HIGH FAT MEAT = 7 GRAMS OF FAT
   AN OUNCE OF LOW FAT MEAT = 3 GRAMS OF FAT

If you think the fat content could be high, count it that way. Otherwise it is probably medium fat unless you know specifics of this product. Be honest on the type of meat, check your list, and your portion and you will see results.

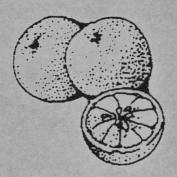

FRUITS AND JUICES

Unsweetened fruits and juices are listed. Double points for sweetened fruit. Avocados have 30 grams fat/avg. fruit. No other fruit or juice contains significant fat to even be considered.

Simple but natural carbohydrates, high in water and fiber and very poorly eaten by much of our society. Use fruits as dessert, appetizers, sweeteners, and fillers, just continue trying different mixtures, different recipes to give your diet variety. Warm fruit is often more flavorful than cold, poached pears, hot apple pie ala mode-fake, and warmed fruit syrups for cereals or waffles are just a few examples.

The darker the color the higher the nutrient content still applies. Check your serving sizes since natural sweetness varies, thus the calories and portions vary as well.

Return to the section on beverages, and you will remember that a small amount of juice is all that is required for vitamins. If you're truly hungry, you need the whole fruit for fiber and filling effect anyway.

Karen's Klue: If you have to eat something, and it's overeating, what better food can you try.

FRUITS AND JUICES

FOOD	AMOUNT	FAT GRAMS	CALORIE PTS	CALORIES
Apple	1 med	0	1	75
Apple Juice	1/2 cup	0	1	75
Applesauce	1/2 cup	0	0.5	37.5
Apricots	4 avg.	0	1	75
Avocado	1 med.	28.5	4.2	315
Banana	1 med.	0	1.5	112.5
Berries:				
Black, Blue, Elder	3/4 cup	0	1	75
Cranberries	1 1/2 cup	0	1	75
Currents, Logan,				
Rasp. & Blueberries	1 cup	0	1	75
Cantaloupe	1/2 med.	0	1	75
Cherries, maraschino	8 lg.	0	1	75
Cherries, red sour	1/2 cup	0	1	75
Cherries, red sweet	15 lg.	0	1	75
Cranberry Juice (lo cal)	3/4 cup	0	1	75
Cranberry Sauce				
(sweetened)	3 T.	0	1	75
Strawberries,				
Gooseberries, and				
Boysenberries	1 1/2 cup	0	1	75
Dates	2 avg.	0	1	75
Fig	1 lg.	0	1	75
Fruit Cocktail	1/2 cup	0	0.5	37.5
Grapes	1/2 cup	0	1.2	90
Grapefruit	1/2 med.	0	5	375
Grapefruit Juice	1/2 cup	0	1	75
Honeydew Melon	1/2 med.	0	1	75
Kiwi	1 1/2 cup	0	1	75
Lemons, Limes	3	0	1	75
Lemon or Lime Juice	1/2 cup	0	0.5	37.5
Mandarin Oranges	1/2 cup	0	1	75
Mango	1/2 med.	0	1	75
Minute Maid Juice:				
Apple	8.45 oz.	0	1.6	120
Berry Punch	8.45 oz.	0	1.7	127.5
Fruit Punch	8.45 oz.	0	1.7	127.5
Orange	8.45 oz.	0	1.6	120
Nectarines	2 med.	0	1	75
Orange	1 med.	0	1	75
Orange Juice	1/2 cup	0	0.5	37.5
Papaya	1 med.	0	1.6	120

FRUITS AND JUICES

FOOD	AMOUNT	FAT GRAMS	CALORIE PTS	CALORIES
Peach	1	0	0.6	45
Peach Slices	1/2 cup	0	0.5	37.5
Peach Nectar	1/2 cup	0	1	75
Pear	1 med.	0	1	75
Pear Nectar	1/2 cup	0	1	75
Pineapple, Fresh	1 cup	0	1	75
Pineapple, Canned	1/2 cup	0	1	75
Pineapple Juice	1/2 cup	0	1	75
Plums	2 med.	0	1	75
Pomegranate	1	0	1	75
Prunes	4 med.	0	1	75
Prune Juice	1/4 cup	0	0.5	37.5
Raisins	2 T.	0	0.5	37.5
Rhubarb, raw	2 cups	0	0.5	37.5
Tangerine	1	0	0.6	45
Watermelon	1 med. wedge	0	1.5	112.5

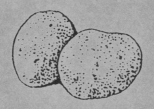

PASTA & RICE

Your refrigerator should contain cooked "grain" at any time. A great high carb staple to add to your snacks or meals, (i.e. cooked pasta, add vegetables and fat free dressing, and small amounts of lean meat for instant meal with fruit and crackers. Bought marinara sauce - home jazzed will make a great Italian style meal with a hard roll and veggie.

Pasta & rice........good at any temp!

Karen's Klue: If you want to increase fiber and begin using whole grains, mix white & wild rice initially, slowly increasing the new higher fiber product, to give your friends and family a chance at liking the tastes!

PASTA AND RICE

ITEM	AMOUNT	FAT GRAMS	CALORIE PTS	CALORIES
Alphabets (Skinner)	2 oz. dry	1	2.7	202.5
DiGiorno				
Angel Hair Pasta	1 cup	2	3.2	240
Cheese Tortelloni	1 cup	6	3.5	262.5
Fettuccini	1 cup	2	3.2	240
Linguini	1 cup	2	3.2	240
Low-Fat Tomato &				
Cheese Tortelloni	1 cup	2	2	150
Egg Noodles				
Martha Gooch	2oz.	3	2.7	202.5
Elbow Macaroni				
(most brands)	2 oz.	1	2.7	202.5
Fettuccini Egg	2 oz.	3	2.7	202.5
Lasagna (Skinner)	2 oz.	1	2.7	202.5
Lasagna Whole Wheat	2 oz.	1	2.7	202.5
Macaroni	2 oz.	1	2.7	202.5
Manicotti	2 oz.	1	2.7	202.5
Mostaccioli	2 oz.	1	2.7	202.5
No Yolk Noodles	1/2 cup	0.5	2.8	210
Reames Free Noodles	1/2 cup	0	2.1	157.5
Rigatoni	2 oz.	1	2.7	202.5
Rotini	2 oz.	1	2.8	210
Spaghetti	2 oz.	1	2.7	202.5
Spaghetti Egg	2 oz.	1	2.7	202.5
Venecia Tortelloni				
all types	2 oz. dry	7	3	225
Vermicelli	2 oz.	1	2.7	202.5
PASTA DINNERS:				
Chef Boyardee- ABC's,				
123's, Dinosaurs, etc.	7.5 oz.	1	2	150
Same Dinners with				
Meatballs	7.5 oz.	11	3.2	240
Kraft Macaroni &				
Cheese	3/4 cup	13	3.7	277.5
Kraft Spaghetti				
w/Meat Sauce Dinner	1cup	14	5	375
Kraft Tangy Italian				
Spaghetti Dinner	1 cup	8	4	300
Lipton Deluxe				
Noodles & Sauce	1/2 cup	10	2	150
Mama Leone's				
Supreme Beef Macaroni	7.5 oz.	7	3.2	240

PASTA AND RICE (continued)

ITEM	AMOUNT	FAT GRAMS	CALORIE PTS	CALORIES
PASTA DINNERS (continued):				
Mama Leone's Spaghetti in Tomato Sauce	7.5 oz.	1	2.2	165
Ragu Pasta Meals:				
Mini Lasagna in Sauce	7.5 oz.	2	2.2	165
Shells in sauce with ground beef	7.5oz.	5	2.5	187.5
PASTA SALAD:				
Betty Crocker Suddenly Salad, Classic Italian	1/2 cup	6	2	150
Lipton:				
Creamy Buttermilk	1/2cup	tr	1.2	90
Garden Macaroni	1/2 cup	tr	1.2	90
Zesty Italian Salad Bar	1/2 cup	5	2	150
Kraft Pasta Salad				
Light Italian	1/2 cup	7	2.5	187.5
Rachers Choice	1/2 cup	16	3.3	247.5
RICE:				
Country Inn Broccoli Rice Au Gratin	1/2 cup	3	2.5	187.5
Country Inn Creamy Mushroom & Wild Rice	1/2 cup	6	2.5	187.5
Kraft Rice & Cheddar Cheese Broccoli	1/2 cup	8	2.5	187.5
Lipton Beef Rice & Sauce	1/2 cup	3	2	150
Lipton Creamy Chicken Rice & Sauce	1/2 cup	8	2.5	187.5
Long Grain Rice	2 oz.	0	1	75
Minute Rice	2/3 cup	2	2	150
Minute Rice Long Grain & Wild Rice	1/2 cup	5	2	150
Natural Brown Rice	1/2 cup	0	1.3	97.5
Uncle Ben Long Grain & Wild Rice	1/2 cup	1	1.3	97.5

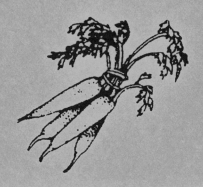

RECIPE INGREDIENTS/CONDIMENTS

This section is a good reminder of the calories and fat contained in some miscellaneous ingredients. When calculating the recipe here are some tips: Add the fat and calories of all ingredients:

Food   Amount   Fat Grams   Calories

Total: fat   calories
Divide number of servings into totals, yet keeping the totals on your recipe assures that you are closer to the actual answer.

Karen's Klue: When changing a recipe for fat and calories, change only one ingredient or preparation method at a time, to understand cause and effect.

RECIPE INGREDIENTS/CONDIMENTS

ITEM	AMOUNT	FAT GRAMS	CALORIE PTS	CALORIES
Baking Chocolate	1 oz.	14.6	2	150
Baking Powder	any	0	0	0
Baking Soda	any	0	0	0
Bouillon	any	0	0	0
Broth, no fat	any	0	0	0
Chocolate Chips, Toll House	1 oz.	8	2	150
Cocoa, Powdered	2 1/2 T.	1	0.5	37.5
Coconut, Bakers Angelflake	1/3 cup	8	1.5	112.5
Coconut, raw	1 oz.	1	1.3	97.5
Condensed Milk Sweetened	1/4 cup	6.6	3	225
Condensed Milk Light Sweetened	2 T.	1.5	1.6	120
Cornstarch	2 1/2 T.	0	1	75
Corn Syrup	1/4 cup	0	3	225
Evaporated Milk Skim	1/2 cup	1	1.5	112.5
Evaporated Milk Whole	1/2 cup	9.5	1.5	112.5
Flour	2 1/2 T.	0	1	75
Gelatin, unflavored	1 env.	0	0.3	22.5
Honey	1 T.	0	1	75
Honey Mustard, Bullseye	2 T.	0	0.8	60
Honey Mustard, KC Masterpiece	2 T.	0	0.6	45
Horseradish	2 T.	0	0	0
Ketchup	2 T.	0	0.5	37.5
Mustard	any	0	0	0
Nuts: Fisher Pecans	1 oz.	19	2.5	187.5
Fisher Walnuts	1 oz.	18	2.5	187.5
Pumpkin Pie Mix, Libby's	1/6 pie	17	5.2	390
Pumpkin, Solid Pack	1/2 cup	0.4	0.5	37.5
Sauces: A-1 Steak Sauce	1 T.	tr	0.2	15
Kikkoman Stir Fry Sauce	1 tsp.	tr	0.2	15
Kikkoman Sweet & Sour Sauce	1 T.	tr	0.2	15

RECIPE INGREDIENTS/CONDIMENTS

ITEM	AMOUNT	FAT GRAMS	CALORIE PTS	CALORIES
Kraft BBQ Sauce	2 T.	1	0.5	37.5
Kraft Fat Free Tarter Sauce	1 T.	0	0.5	37.5
Kraft Hickory Smoke BBQ	2 T.	1	0.5	37.5
Kraft Tarter Sauce	1 T.	8	1	75
La Choy Teriyaki Marinade	1 oz.	0	1.5	112.5
Open Pit BBQ Sauce Hickory Sauceworks Sweet & Sour	1 T.	0	0.2	15
INGREDIENTS:				
Seasonings:				
Salt, Pepper, Most Herbs & Spices	any	0	0	0
Sugar:				0
Brown	2 T.	0	1.5	112.5
Powdered & White	2 T.	0	1	75
White, lump	3 small	0	1	75
Syrups:				
Corn, sorghum	1 1/2 T.	0	1	75
Maple	1 1/2 T.	0	1	75
Maple, diet	1/4 cup	0	0	0
Molasses, light	2 T.	0	1	75
Vinegar	any	0	0	0
Yeast, Brewers	2 T.	0	0.5	37.5

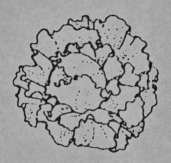

SALAD BAR, SOUP, AND VEGETABLES

Whatever you like, try to find new ways to prepare, and new ingredients to accompany. We should truly never get tired of these carbohydrate, and high fiber sources that taste very different from each other.

Of course homemade soups are the flavor feasts and the hearty comfort foods that you might choose first. Keep watching for natural chicken bases, pasta vegetable soups, any products that you can enjoy as they are or with a few added ingredients of your own.

Other countries truly don't understand the low intake of vegetables, and soups that America exists on. Order these as appetizers or snacks whenever possible. If you are eating 4-6 times daily, these foods keep the athlete of any sport or interest mentally and physically prepared.

Karen's Klue: A hot soup is filling, as if you had high quantity or high fiber. It slows down the eating process and is a good rule of thumb for slowing down intake of calories overall.

SALAD BAR, SOUP, VEGETABLES

ITEM	AMOUNT	FAT GRAMS	CALORIE PTS	CALORIES
Alfalfa	1 T.	4.5	0.6	45
Bacon Bits	2 T.	7.2	2	150
Bean Sprouts	1/2 cup	0	2.5	187.5
Beets	1/4 cup	0	0.5	37.5
Broccoli	1/2 cup	0	0.2	15
Carrots	strips	0	0	0
Cauliflower	3/4 cup	0	0.2	15
Celery	any	0	0	0
Cherry Tomatoes	5	0	0.7	52.5
Cottage Cheese, 4%	1/2 cup	4.75	1.5	112.5
Croutons	3 T.	3	0.6	45
Cucumber	0.5	0	0.2	15
Grated Cheese	1 T.	4.5	0.6	45
Grated Egg	1/2 egg	4	0.5	37.5
Green Onions	12	0	0.2	15
Green Pepper	strips	0	0	0
Fresh Fruit Salad	1/2 cup	0	1	75
Hot Peppers	6	0	0.2	15
Macaroni Salad	1/2 cup	12.8	1.5	112.5
Mixed Greens	any	0	0	0
Potato Salad	1/2 cup	10.3	1.5	112.5
Radish	any	0	0	0
Raisins	2 T.	0	1	75
Sunflower Seeds	1 oz.	16	2.2	165
Sweet Pickle Chips	6	0	1	75
Starchy Vegetables	1/2 cup	0	1	75
Carrots, Beets, Onion, Peas	1/2 cup	0	0.5	37.5
All other Vegetables	1/2 cup	0	0	0

The following vegetables are listed as prepared without butter,margarine, or sauces added:

Alfalfa sprouts	1/2 cup	0	0.5	37.5
Artichoke	1 lg. bud	0	0.5	37.5
Artichoke Hearts	1/2 cup	0	0.5	37.5
Asparagus	1 cup	0	0.5	37.5
Avocado, CA. or FL.	1 med.	30	4	300
Bamboo Shoots	1 1/4 cup	0	0.5	37.5
Beans, Green or Wax	1 cup	0	0.5	37.5
Bean Sprouts	1 cup	0	0.5	37.5
Beets	1/2 cup	0	0.5	37.5
Broccoli	1 cup	0	0.5	37.5

SALAD BAR, SOUP, VEGETABLES

ITEM	AMOUNT	FAT GRAMS	CALORIE PTS	CALORIES

The following vegetables are listed as prepared without butter, margarine, or sauces added (continued):

ITEM	AMOUNT	FAT GRAMS	CALORIE PTS	CALORIES
Brussel Sprouts	3/4 cup	0	0.5	37.5
Cabbage, cooked	1 cup	0	0.5	37.5
Cabbage, raw, shredded	2 cups	0	0.5	37.5
Carrots	1/2 cup	0	0.5	37.5
Carrots with br. sugar	1/2 cup	0	1	75
Cauliflower	1 1/2 cup	0	0.5	37.5
Celery	8 8" stalks	0	0.5	37.5
Chard	3/4 cup	0	0.5	37.5
Chick Peas	1/2 cup	2	1.8	135
Coleslaw	1/2 cup	0	1	75
Collards	3/4 cup	0	0.5	37.5
Corn, Cream Style	3/4 cup	0	1.5	112.5
Corn on the Cob	1 med	0	0.5	37.5
Corn, Whole Kernel	1/2 cup	0	1	75
Cucumber	1 med	0	0.5	37.5
Dandelion Greens	1/2 cup	0	0.5	37.5
Eggplant	3/4 cup	0	0.5	37.5
Endive	40 leaves	0	0.5	37.5
Escarole	8 lg. leaves	0	0.5	37.5
Garbanzo Beans	1/2 cup	2	1.8	135
Hominy	1/2 cup	0	1	75
Kale	1 cup	0	0.5	37.5
Kidney Beans	1/2 cup	0.5	1.5	112.5
Kohlrabi	1 cup	0	0.5	37.5
Leeks	1/2 cup	0	0.5	37.5
Lettuce (med. head)	1	0	1	75
Lettuce, shredded	1/2 cup	0	0.1	7.5
Mixed Vegetables	3/4 cup	0	1	75
Mushrooms	3/4 cup	0	0.5	37.5
Mustard Greens	1 cup	0	1	75
Okra	12	0	0.5	37.5
Onion	1/2 cup	0	0.5	37.5
Onion, Green	12 small	0	0.5	37.5
Parsnips	2/3 cup	0	1	75
Peas, green	1/2 cup	0	0.5	37.5
Peppers, hot chili	1	0	0.2	15
Peppers, jalapeno	1/2 cup	0	0.2	15
Peppers, sweet	1/2 cup	0	0.2	15
Pimento	6 med.	0	0.5	37.5

SALAD BAR, SOUP, VEGETABLES

ITEM	AMOUNT	FAT GRAMS	CALORIE PTS	CALORIES

The following vegetables are listed as prepared without butter, margarine, or sauces added:

ITEM	AMOUNT	FAT GRAMS	CALORIE PTS	CALORIES
Potato 1 sm, 3/4 med, 1/2 lg.	1	0	1	75
Potato, mashed plain	1/2 cup	0	1	75
Potato, mashed with butter & milk	1/2 cup	10	1.5	112.5
Potato, scalloped or creamed	1/2 cup	10	1.5	112.5
Pumpkin	1/2 cup	0	0.5	37.5
Radishes	any	0	0	0
Rhubarb	1 cup	0	0.3	22.5
Rutabega	1/2 cup	0	0.5	37.5
Sauerkraut	3/4 cup	0	0.5	37.5
Snow Peas	3 oz.	0	0.4	30
Spinach	3/4 cup	0	0.5	37.5
Squash, Summer: Banana, Crookneck, Scallop, Straight Neck, Zucchini	1 cup	0	0.5	37.5
Squash, Winter: Acorn, Buttercup, Butternut, Hubbard	1 cup	0	0.5	37.5
Sweet Potato or Yam	1/2 med.	0	1	75
Sweet Potato or Yam Candied	3/4 cup	0	4	300
Three-Bean Salad	2/5 cup	0	1	75
Tomato	1/2 med	0	1	75
Tomato, cooked	3/4 cup	0	0.5	37.5
Tomato Juice	3/4 cup	0	0.5	37.5
Tomato Paste	1 1/2 oz.	0	0.5	37.5
Tomato Puree	6 T.	0	0.5	37.5
Tomato Sauce	1/2 cup	0	0.5	37.5
Turnips	1 cup	0	0.5	37.5
Turnip Greens	1 1/2 cup	0	1	75
Vegetable Juice Cocktail	3/4 cup	0	0.5	37.5

SALAD BAR, SOUP, VEGETABLES

ITEM	AMOUNT	FAT GRAMS	CALORIE PTS	CALORIES
SOUPS:				
Borscht	1 cup	5	0	0
Campbells Healthy Requests:				
Bean w/Bacon	1 cup	4	2	150
Chicken Noodle	1 cup	2	1	75
Chicken w/Rice	1 cup	2	1	75
Cream of Chicken	1 cup	2	1	75
Cream of Mushroom	1 cup	2	1	75
Campbells Healthy Requests prepared according to directions:				
Cream of Broccoli	8 oz.	2	1.3	97.5
Cream of Celery	8 oz.	2	1.3	97.5
Healthy Vegetable	8 oz.	1	1.2	90
Split Pea	8 oz.	2	2	150
Tomato Vegetable	8 oz.	2	1.7	127.5
Vegetable Beef	8 oz.	2	1	75
Campbell Chunky Soups, ready to eat:				
Chicken Noodle	9.2 oz.	5.5	2.1	157.5
Chicken w/Rice	9.5 oz.	3.8	1.8	135
Ham n' Bean	9.6 oz.	7.8	3.2	240
Minestrone	7.3 oz.	2.1	0.9	67.5
New England Style	9.5 oz.	14.8	3.3	247.5
Pepper Steak	10.8 oz.	2.6	2.3	172.5
Sirloin Burger	9.5 oz.	7.5	2.5	187.5
Steak & Potato	10.5 oz.	5	2.7	202.5
Dehydrated Soup Mix:				
Chicken Noodle	1 cup	0.5	0.5	37.5
Onion	1 cup	0.5	0.5	37.5
Dehydrated Single Serving Soups:				
Broth Type	1 cup	0.5	0.5	37.5
Cream Type	1 cup	2 to 4	1	75
Campbells:				
Beef Flavor Noodle	1 pkg.	2	1.8	135
Chicken flavor	1 pkg.	1.5	2.9	217.5
Knorr:				
Black Bean	1 pkg.	1	2.6	195
Chicken Vegetable	1 pkg.	0	1.3	97.5
Potato Leek	1 pkg.	0	1.6	120

SALAD BAR, SOUP, VEGETABLES

ITEM	AMOUNT	FAT GRAMS	CALORIE PTS	CALORIES
Canned, condensed (prepared w/equal amount of whole milk):				
Clam Chowder	1 cup	14	3	225
Cream of Chicken or Celery	1 cup	9.7	2.5	187.5
Cream of Mushroom	1 cup	9.7	2.5	187.5
Cream Of Tomato	1 cup	6	2.6	195
Canned, condensed (prepared with equal amount of water):				
Bean with Pork & Bean	1 cup	5.9	2.5	187.5
Beef or Chicken Bouillon	any	0	0	0
Beef or Chicken Noodle	1 cup	2.5	1	75
Clam Chowder, New				0
England	1 cup	3.1	1.6	120
Cream of Chicken/				0
Celery	1 cup	7.4	1.5	112.5
Cream of Mushroom	1 cup	7.2	2	150
Cream of Tomato	1 cup	1.9	1	75
Split Pea	1 cup	4.4	2	150
Tomato	1 cup	2	1	75
Vegetable Beef	1 cup	1.9	1	75
Vegetarian Vegetable	1 cup	0	1	75
Tomato w/skim milk	1 cup	2	2	150
Ready to Serve Varieties:				
Chicken Broth	1 cup	0	0.2	15
Hearty Chicken Noodle	1 cup	2	1	75
Hearty Chicken & Rice	1 cup	2	1.5	112.5
Hearty Chicken & Vegetable	1 cup	2	1.5	112.5
Hearty Minestrone	1 cup	2	1	75
Hearty Vegetable	1 cup	1	1	75
Hearty Vegetable Beef	1 cup	3	1.5	112.5
Vegetable Beef	1 cup	2	1	75
Health Valley Brand Soups:				
Chili w/Black Beans	5 oz.	0	2	150
Country Corn & Veg.	1 cup	0	1	75
Five Bean Vegetable	1 cup	0	1.3	97.5
14 Garden Vegetable	1 cup	0	0.75	56.25

SALAD BAR, SOUP, VEGETABLES

ITEM	AMOUNT	FAT GRAMS	CALORIE PTS	CALORIES
Health Valley Brand Soups (continued):				
Italian Minestrone	1 cup	0	1	75
Tomato Vegetable	1 cup	0	0.7	52.5
Vegetable Barley	1 cup	0	1	75
Home Made Soups:				
Bean with Ham	3/4 cup	8.5	3.3	247.5
Beef Barley	1/2 cup	1.4	1.3	97.5
Cauliflower, creamed	1/2 cup	9.7	1.6	120
Celery, creamed	3/4 cup	9.7	2	150
Corn Chowder	1/2 cup	12	1.6	120
Oyster Stew (1 pt. oyster, 2 pt. whole milk)	1/2 cup	10	1.3	97.5
Vegetable Beef	1 cup	4	1.5	112.5
Vegetable soup	1 cup	1	1	75
Progresso Pasta Soups:				
Hearty Chicken &				0
Rotini	1 cup	2	1.2	90
Hearty Minestrone &				0
Shells	1 cup	1.5	1.6	120
Hearty Penne	9.5 oz.	1	1	75
Hearty Tomato &				
Rotini	1 cup	5	1.6	120
Hearty Veg. & Rotini	1 cup	1	1.4	105
Meatballs & Pasta				
Pearls	1 cup	7	1.8	135
Soup Starter:				
Beef Barley	1 serving	0.5	1.3	97.5
Beef Vegetable	1 serving	0.5	1.2	90
Chicken Noodle	1 serving	0.5	1	75
Ground Beef Veg.	1 serving	0.5	1	75

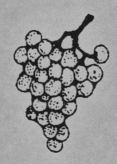

NEBRASKA'S CHOICE RESTAURANTS

In Nebraska there are restaurants willing and asking to have menu items caluculated for your benefit. They want to provide you more information on the best choices for your health and your enjoyment. We are fortunate to add to this edition a new list of "AFARES" of the Heart", a program by registered dietitians at Omaha Methodists' nutrition department working with Omaha and Lincoln restaurants. Their healthy heart entrees meet the criteria of fat and calories set by the hospital program.

Karen's Klue: **ASK QUESTIONS>>>>**Be sure to ask how sauces and extras are prepared, any recipe items, and to let the waiter know you want to hear the low fat, and heart healthy specials....Remember you are the expert though, the staff may not have had as much training as you in selecting choices with fat and calories savings.... so "on the side" with any questionable extras is smart planning.

COUNTRY KITCHEN

ITEM	AMOUNT	FAT GRAMS	CALORIE PTS	CALORIES
Blueberry Pancakes*	1 order	12	4.2	315
Cold Cereal & Fruit	1 order	5	5.7	427.5
Granola & Fruit	1 order	7.5	3.3	247.5
Pancakes*	Full Stack	11.5	5.2	390
Pancakes*	Short Stack	9.5	4.5	337.5

*Meets Right Choice guidelines without breakfast meat

ITEM	AMOUNT	FAT GRAMS	CALORIE PTS	CALORIES
Grilled Chicken Sandwich**	1	21	7	525
French Dip**	1	19	8.5	637.5

**Meets Right Choice guidelines without french fries

ITEM	AMOUNT	FAT GRAMS	CALORIE PTS	CALORIES
Chicken Teriyaki***	1 dinner	22	9.5	712.5
Grilled Chicken***	1 dinner	28	10.75	806.25
Smothered Chicken***	1 dinner	28.5	11	825
Senior Grilled Chicken***	1 dinner	13.5	5.5	412.5

***Meets Right Choice guidelines when served with rice pilaf, whipped or
  baked potato

You can make the "RIGHT CHOICE" at Country Kitchen.
Country Kitchen takes the guess work out of healthful dining. Their unique
"Right Choice Program assures you that the choices are under 30% fat. The
staff aim to please, so ask questions, study the menu possibilities, and enjoy
soon.

DRIESBACH'S

ITEM	AMOUNT	FAT GRAMS	CALORIE PTS	CALORIES
APPETIZERS & SALADS:				
Lite Relish Plate	1 order	0	0.5	37.5
Shrimp Cocktails	3 oz. order	1	1	75
Lite Chef Salad	1 order	11	3.3	247.5
	1 order	15	4	300
	1 order	16.5	4	300
Green Vegetables	1/2 cup	0	0	0
Corn	1/2 cup	0	1	75
Italian Caper Dressing	1 T.	7	1	75
Dinner Salad Regular	regular	0	0.5	37.5
SIDE ORDERS:				
Baked Potato	8 oz.	0	3	225
Vegetable Soup	2 cups	0	1	75
RicePilaf	1/2 cup	0	1	75
ENTREES:				
Broiled Shrimp	5 shrimp	1	1	75
Ground Beef Steak	5 oz.	10.6	4.3	322.5
Tenderloin Steak	5 1/2 oz.	14.4	4.2	315
Marinated Chicken				
Breast	4 oz.	3	1.75	131.25
Halibut	5 oz.	4	2.6	195
Scallops	5 oz.	2	2	150
Trout	6 oz.	7.3	3.3	247.5
Orange Roughy	8 oz.	15	3.7	277.5
King Salmon	6 oz.	12.8	4	300

Great changes are continuing at Dreisbach's. We've given you the basics, but with time they will be offering even more entrees and side dishes prepared low in fat. Pat Dowd and his staff will honor your requests and try to help you eat a meal to enjoy, from lean beef to a variety of fish and poultry, with fresh side dishes to complement the effect. Get back to Dreisbach's soon.... heart healthy dining!

FARMER'S DAUGHTER

ITEM	AMOUNT	FAT GRAMS	CALORIE PTS	CALORIES
BREAKFAST:				
Egg	1	6	1.0	75
Toast w/o butter	2 slices	2	2.0	150
Sugar free jelly	1 Tbs.	0	0.3	20
Cinnamon roll	1	13.8	6.3	474
Danish Pastry	1	17	4.0	300
English Muffin				
w/o butter	1	2	2.0	150
Bagel	1	3.5	2.8	210
Pancake	1	1.75	1.5	116
Short Stack	2	3.5	3.1	232
Stack of Cakes	3	5.25	4.6	348
Bacon	3 strips	9.4	1.5	110
Sausage	2 patties	16	2.7	200
Sausage	3 links	12.3	1.9	144
Ham	2 oz.	3	1.1	81
Ham	3 oz.	5	1.6	122
Oatmeal w/1% milk	1 cup	3.5	3.3	245
Oatmeal w/1% milk	1 bowl	5.8	5.2	390
Cold Cereal				
Wheaties	1 cup	1	1.5	112
Rice Krispies	1 cup	0	1.5	112
Special K	1 cup	0	1.5	112
Raisin Bran	2/3 cup	1	1.7	125
Frosted Flakes	3/4 cup	0	1.5	112
with 1% milk		2.5	1.3	100
Grapefruit	1/2	0	0.5	40
Cantaloupe	1 1/2 cup	0	1.1	85
French Toast	2	3	3.0	223
Hot Chocolate	1 cup	3	1.3	98
Juice				
Orange	6 oz.	0	0.7	56
Apple	6 oz.	0	1.5	112
Orange	12 oz.	0	1.0	75
Apple	12 oz.	0	2.0	150
Chocolate Milk	8 oz.	2.5	2.1	158
OTHER DISHES:				
Chef Salad w/o				
dressing (small)	1	12.5	3.1	230
Chef Salad w/o				
dressing (large)	1	25	5.7	430
Combination Salad	1 cup	0	0.3	20
Lettuce Salad	1 cup	0	0.2	18

FARMER'S DAUGHTER (continued)

ITEM	AMOUNT	FAT GRAMS	CALORIE PTS	CALORIES
Fat Free Buttermilk				
Dressing	1.5 oz.	0	0.6	45
Diet Center Dressing	2 tsp.	10.5	1.3	96
Cottage Cheese	1/2 cup	2	1.3	98
Salad Plate				
(lettuce salad in place				
of potato salad)				
w/beef & crackers	1	8.2	4.2	318
w/chicken & crackers	1	5.5	3.2	243
w/ham & crackers	1	8.5	4.0	298
w/tuna & crackers	1	4.5	3.7	280
Diet Plate w/crackers	1	7.2	5.4	406
DC Chef Salad				
w/o DC Dressing	1	8.6	3.3	245
DC Chicken Salad				
DC Mayo				
lowfat dressing	1	7.6	3.2	243
fat free dressing	1	3.6	3.1	233
SOUP:				
Beef Barley	1 cup	1.46	0.7	58
Beef Barley	bowl	2.92	1.5	116
Chicken Noodle	1 cup	2	0.9	71
Chicken Noodle	bowl	4	1.9	142
Chili	1 cup	8	2.5	187
Chili	bowl	16	5	374
Ham & Bean	1 cup	1	0.4	30
Ham & Bean	bowl	2	0.8	60
Potato	1 cup	9	1.4	106
Potato	bowl	18	2.8	212
Vegetable	1 cup	2	0.7	50
Vegetable	bowl	4	1.4	100
DC Pie	1 piece	3	1.4	108
DC Muffin	1	2.75	0.9	70
DINNERS:				
Roast Beef w/o soup				
& added butter	1	18	9.2	687
Hamburger Steak w/o				
soup or added butter	1	23.5	10.7	805
Hot Beef w/potatoes				
& gravy	1	14	7.0	524
Corn Beef Sandwich				
w/o added sauce or				
dressing	1	36.3	7.2	538

FARMER'S DAUGHTER (continued)

ITEM	AMOUNT	FAT GRAMS	CALORIE PTS	CALORIES
French Dip Sandwich w/o french fries	1	15	6.7	505
Roast Beef Sandwich request w/o dressing w/o chips)	1	11	3.7	275
Ham & Cheese w/o chips, request w/o dressing)	1	13.7	4.2	318
Bacon 3 slices, lettuce tomato w/o chips request w/o dressing	1	11.3	3.4	257.72

At the Farmer's Daugher Cafe we take great pride in our outstanding home cooked food, and quick and friendly tableservice. We offer a wide variety of foods to satisfy any appetite. Many menu items are low in fat, and calories. We prepare special orders, JUST ASK.....

Our smoke free dining promotes a healthy atmosphere. Open M-F 6 a.m.- 3p.m. and 7a.m.-11a.m. on Saturday . Join us soon....

GARDEN CAFE, HASTINGS

ITEM	AMOUNT	FAT GRAMS	CALORIE PTS	CALORIES
Heart Fruit Plate				
w/low fat muffin	1	2	6.8	508
w/bran muffin	1	12	7.2	538
Heart French Toast				
w/applesauce	1	3	4.3	324
w/low cal syrup	1	3	4.9	368
Heart Omelet				
w/fruit	1	2	3	227
w/lowfat muffin	1	2	5	375
w/bran muffin	1	12	5.4	405
Heart Chicken Stirfry				
w/lowfat muffin	1	5	5.9	445
w/bran muffin	1	14	6.3	475
w/dinner roll	1	6	3.7	280
Heart Italian Chicken				
w/rice	1	6	6.3	473
Polynesian Chicken				
w/rice	1	3	6.2	464
Heart Halibut Dinner				
w/rice	1	6	5.5	410
Heart Potato Casserole				
w/lowfat muffin	1	12	9.4	702
w/bran muffin	1	21	9.8	732
w/dinner roll	1	13	7.2	538
Heart Jacket Potato				
w/fruit	1	12	5.8	433
Heart Salad w/Dole Whip				
& lowfat muffin	1	8	6.6	493
& bran muffin	1	17	7	523
& dinner roll	1	10	4.4	328
Heart Spinach Salad				
w/lowfat muffin	1	5	5.4	408
w/bran muffin	1	14	5.8	438
w/dinner roll	1	7	3.3	244
Heart Chef Salad				
w/lowfat muffin	1	10	7.3	551
w/bran muffin	1	19	7.7	581
w/dinner roll	1	12	5.1	386

GARDEN CAFE, HASTINGS (continued)

ITEM	AMOUNT	FAT GRAMS	CALORIE PTS	CALORIES
Heart French Dip w/fruit	1	7	4.5	335
Heart Chicken Sand. w/fruit	1	16	6.8	512
Heart Melt w/fruit	1	10	4.4	330

The restaurant Central Nebraska has been waiting for. One look at the menu and its clear that The Garden Cafe is ready to please all of its customers with selections ranging from their famous potato casserole, to the great and even lean sandwiches.

A wedge of fruits is a normal garnish to add to your meal, with fresh baked muffins and breads waiting to melt-in -your mouth.....So drive to the Garden for a colorful fun experience any time of day....

GRAND ISLAND WEST
ALDA 76 RESTAURANT

ITEM	AMOUNT	FAT GRAMS	CALORIE PTS	CALORIES
Pancakes, Stack	3 cakes	23.5	7.5	562.5
Pancakes, Short Stack	2 cakes	15.5	5	375
Chicken Noodle Soup	1 cup	3	2	150
Beef Noodle Soup	1 cup	4	3.6	274.5
Vegetable Soup	1 cup	2	1.7	131
Chef Salad	1	16	4.3	322.5
Chef Salad w/o Egg	1	11	3.3	247.5
French Dip				
Sandwich only	1	12.5	4.2	319
Coleslaw	1/2 cup	5	2.5	187.5
Spaghetti (Entree only)	1 order	12	7.2	544
Meatloaf	5 oz.	26	5	375

Good home cooking is what you will get when you stop by Alda 76. Everything is homemade, and delicious. They have several power foods on their menu that you can be assured are healthy and within the guidelines for heart healthy lifestyles.Two percent milk is available along with light dressing. Feel free to enjoy their old fashioned hospitality while staying healthy.

GRANDMA MAX'S

ITEM	AMOUNT	FAT GRAMS	CALORIE PTS	CALORIES
LITE BREAKFAST:				
Hot Cereal	4 oz.	5	4.3	320
Lite Pancakes	3	0	2.4	181
LITE DINNER: with *baked potato, fat free sour cream, salad & fat free salad dressing				
Top Sirloin	1 serving	9.72	8.3	622
Roast Turkey	1 serving	0.2	5.4	404
Broiled Halibut	1 serving	5.2	7.4	552
*Averages with brown rice or mixed vegetables:				
	1 serving	+.87	-1.1	-80
LITE LUNCHES: with *baked potato & fat free sour cream				
Chicken Philly Sand.	1	1.2	7.5	561
Light Club Sandwich	1	17.2	9.8	737.4
Light Cheeseburger	1	13.5	7.7	577
Turkey Sandwich	1	1.8	6.1	454
*Changes with fruit instead of baked potato				
	1	-0.2	-1.7	-126
LITE DESSERTS:				
Light Apple Pie	1 serving	8	3.5	262
Fruit Bowl	1 serving	0	1.7	124
Fresh Fruit	1 serving	0	1.3	100
OTHER SIDE DISHES:				
Steamed Mixed Vegetables	1 serving	0.8	1.6	118
Steamed Br. Rice	1 serving	1.35	2.2	162
Tossed Salad with fat free dressing	1 serving	0	0.9	64
Fat Free Sour Cream	2 T.	0	0.4	30
Chili	6 oz.	9.5	2.7	205
Chili	10.oz	19	5.5	411
Muffins				
Blueberry	3 oz.	10	4.7	354
Banana	3 oz.	12	5.7	428
Oatbran	3 oz.	14	5.8	433
Yogurt, Lite & Lively	6 oz.	0	2.3	170

GRANDMA MAX'S (continued)

ITEM	AMOUNT	FAT GRAMS	CALORIE PTS	CALORIES
BEVERAGES				
Skim Milk	8 oz.	0.4	1.1	86
Juice				
Orange	4 oz.	0.1	0.7	56
Tomato	4 oz.	0	0.3	25
Grapefruit	4 oz.	0.1	0.6	46
Coffee	8 oz.	0	0.1	4

Grandma Max's- is well known for their fine quality Restaurant. The meats and other ingredients are second to none. Real mashed potatoes are always available, and with a new "Light" menu the choices are well planned, and tested, for popularity and health. Any time of day, check our list of Grandma Max's healthy selections, and then consider that low fat, no sugar cherry pie, just before heading home.....Just like Grandma's.

HABE'TAT

ITEM	AMOUNT	FAT GRAMS	CALORIE PTS	CALORIES
Wild Rice Soup	1 cup	15	3.2	240
Thin Crust Pizza	1/2 pizza	13.75	5.2	390
Tossed Salad	1 order	0.5	1.5	112.5
Caesar Salad	1 order	8.75	3.2	240
Grilled Chicken Salad	1 order	5	4	300
French Dip	1	20	8	600
Grilled Chicken Sandwich	1	18	8.5	637.5
Filet (7 oz. before grilling)	1	16	4.7	356.2
Light Italian Dressing	1 T.	3	0.5	37.5

NEW MENU COMING SOON....
ALONG WITH THESE GREAT TRADITIONALS !!!

We've listed just a few of the great traditionals that will continue at Habe'tat. Since the word is out when their new menu with more great choices will be in. You will want to assume only that this is just a beginning of gourmet foods that Habe'tat will continue offering , and a great reason to dine their soon. Special requests are honored when possible.

HUNAN'S

ITEM	AMOUNT	FAT GRAMS	CALORIE PTS	CALORIES
Egg Roll	1	10	2	150
Wanton	1	10	1.5	112.5
Sauces:				
White	1 cup	3	1	75
Brown	1 cup	3	1	75
Sweet & Sour	1/2 cup	0	1.5	112.5
Soy Sauce	1/4 cup	0	0.6	45
Soups:				
Egg Drop	1 serving	4	0.5	37.5
Wanton Soup	1 serving	1	0.5	37.5
Spicy Sour	1 serving	1	1	75
Fried Rice	1 cup	7	3	225

*All entrees are figured without sauce and rice:

ITEM	AMOUNT	FAT GRAMS	CALORIE PTS	CALORIES
Lobster Shrimp Dinner	1	2.5	3.5	262.5
Triple Delight Dinner	1	9	4.2	319
Princess Chicken &				
Shrimp Dinner	1	11.75	3.75	281
Lunch Entree	1	11	3	225
Scallops & Beef Dinner	1	10	4.5	337.5
Lake Tung Ting Shrimp				
Dinner	1	5	3.3	250
Happy Family Dinner	1	11.75	5.5	412.5
Moo Goo Gai Pan				
Dinner	1	6.5	4.5	337.5
Lunch entree	1	4.5	3.2	244
Sliced Chicken sauted				with
Broccoli Dinner	1	6.5	4.5	337.5
Lunch Entree	1	4.5	3	225
Hunan Shrimp Dinner	1	2.5	3.2	244
Lunch Entree	1	2	2.5	187.5
Hunan Pork Dinner	1	19.75	5.2	394
Lunch Entree	1	14	3.7	281
Shredded Pork with				
Garlic Sauce Dinner	1	19.25	4.7	356
Lunch Entree	1	14.5	3.5	262.5
Pepper Steak Dinner	1	15	4.7	356
Lunch Entree	1	13.25	4.7	300

HUNAN'S (continued)

ITEM	AMOUNT	FAT GRAMS	CALORIE PTS	CALORIES
Sliced Beef with				
Broccoli Dinner	1	17.5	5.5	412.5
Lunch Entree	1	12	3.7	281
Shredded Beef				
Szechwan Style Dinner	1	14.5	4.5	337.5
Steamed Dumpling				
Dinner	1	10.4	4.3	322.5
Fried Dumpling Dinner	1	16	5.2	390

Hunan's use the freshest ingredients available. Their meat is the leanest you can buy. Lean Beef flank steaks and chicken breasts are just a few of the quality cuts included in their preparation. Regular rice is available for anyone desiring to keep their fat grams lower. Stop in soon for a luncheon or dinner meal to enjoy.

IMPERIAL PALACE EXPRESS

ITEM	AMOUNT	FAT GRAMS	CALORIE PTS	CALORIES
Almond Chicken	1	24.4	6.9	520
Snow White Chicken	1	8.6	4.0	300
Sweet & Sour Chicken	1	17	8.0	600
Princess Chicken	1	32.4	8.7	650
Broccoli Chicken	1	8.66	4.0	300
Broccoli Beef	1	26.7	6.4	482
Pepper Beef	1	32	7.3	548
Sweet & Sour Pork	1	26.9	8.1	604
Hot Braised Pork	1	47.9	12.0	902
Vegetable Deluxe	1	5.2	2.6	192
Chicken Chow Mein	1	20.9	6.3	471
Beef Chow Mein	1	22.2	6.3	475
Cashew Chicken	1	33.1	7.0	525
Imperial Chicken	1	17.5	7.5	560
Lemon Chicken	1	17.5	6.2	462
Mongolian Beef	1	26.8	7.2	539
Kung Pao Beef	1	49.3	8.9	666.5
Lemon Shrimp	1	16.4	6.0	452
Imperial Shrimp	1	21	7.9	590
Shrimp w/vegetables	1	6	3.1	234
Sweet & Sour Shrimp	1	22.5	7.2	539
Kung Pao Shrimp	1	6.5	3.4	258
Three Delicacies	1	12.7	4.5	339
Chicken Fried Rice	2 1/2 cup	16.4	12.6	945
Shrimp Fried Rice	2 1/2 cup	6.6	9.6	720
Beef Fried Rice	2 1/2 cup	17.4	11.8	882
Cashew Chicken w/ boiled chicken	1	16.2	5.2	391
Imperial Chicken w/ boiled chicken	1	8.5	6.4	480
Lemon Chicken w/ boiled chicken	1	8.4	5.1	381
Kung Pao Chicken w/boiled chicken	1	6.5	3.4	258
Hot & Sour Soup	8 oz.	2	0.8	60
Hot & Sour Soup	12 oz.	3	1.2	91
Egg Drop Soup	8 oz.	2	0.8	57
Egg Drop Soup	12 oz.	3	1.1	84
Imperial Sauce	1 cup	0.1	2.5	190
Lemon Sauce	1 cup	0	1.3	98
Brown Sauce	1 cup	0.8	3.1	236

IMPERIAL PALANCE EXPRESS (continued)

ITEM	AMOUNT	FAT GRAMS	CALORIE PTS	CALORIES
White Sauce	1 cup	0.1	0.1	10
Hot Braised Sauce	1 cup	0.18	1.8	138
Sweet & Sour Sauce	1 cup	0	2.1	160
Marinated Dark Chicken	3.5 oz.	11.6	4.3	325
Marinated White Chicken	3.5 oz.	5	2.7	200
Marinated Shrimp	3.5 oz.	2.7	1.8	134
Marinated Beef	3.5 oz.	12.6	3.5	262

Imperial Palace Express at the Conestoga Mall in Grand Island has a great menu of Chinese entrees and side dishes that can easily be diversified. The folks at Imperial Palace are more than willing to add boiled shrimp or boiled chicken to their already healthy entrees. The staff will serve you a generous portion of vegetables and meat combined with a tasty sauce. Keep Imperial Palace in mind for a great meal while shopping.

INCREDIBLE BULK, THE

ITEM	AMOUNT	FAT GRAMS	CALORIE PTS	CALORIES
Asher's Sugar Free candies w/ milk chocolate flavored coating:				
Almond Bark	2 pieces	15	2.7	200
Cashew Clusters	4 pieces	16	2.8	210
Cherry Nut Nougat	4 pieces	9	1.9	140
Chocolate Fudge Meltaway	3 pieces	16	2.7	200
Coconut Clusters	4 pieces	22	3.6	270
Coconut Royale Cream	3 pieces	11	2.3	170
Cordial Cherry	3 pieces	6	1.9	140
Mint Truffle	3 pieces	10	2.3	170
Peanut Butter Cups	1 cup	16	2.7	200
Peanut Clusters	4 pieces	17	2.8	210
Peanut Truffle	3 pieces	16	2.7	200
Pecan Caramel Pattie	2 pieces	15	2.9	220
Raspberry Sherbert Creams	2 pieces	8	2.0	150
Vanilla Butter Creams	3 pieces	8	1.9	140
Vanilla Caramels	3 pieces	11	2.8	210
Cocoa Amore Sugar-Free Hot Chocolate:				
Choc. Raspberry	8 oz.	5	1.2	90
Choc. Supreme	8 oz.	5	1.2	90
Irish Cream	8 oz.	5	1.2	90
Georgia Nut Co.:				
Sugar Free Milk Ch. Flavored Almonds	10 pieces	18	3.2	240
Go Lightly:				
Sugar Free Fruit Chews	7 pieces	1.5	2.1	160
Sugar Free Caramels	5 pieces	6	2.5	190
Sugar Free Chocolate Crunch	7 pieces	13	3.1	230
Sugar Free Fudgie Rolls	6 pieces	4.5	2.3	170

INCREDIBLE BULK (continued)

ITEM	AMOUNT	FAT GRAMS	CALORIE PTS	CALORIES

Goelitz Sugar-Free Candies include:
Gummy Bears, Jelly Beans, Red Licorice,
Black Licorice, Starlight Mints

Golden Batch Sugar-Free Wafers in:
Chocolate, Vanilla & Peanut Butter

The nutritional information is unavailable at this time.

At Incredible Bulk, Gayle is always finding new candies to give you choices. He has found low fat and low sugar candies that benefit all of us.....with great taste. Come in and try some of the products listed. Then you'll want to spread the news to people with diabetes, cardiac, and weight concerns.You won't know the variety you can have without guilt feelings.....till you try.

INTERSTATE HOLIDAY INN

ITEM	AMOUNT	FAT GRAMS	CALORIE PTS	CALORIES
BREAKFAST:				
Pancakes	2	6	3	225
Belgian waffle	1	6	2.3	173
1 Cholesterol-free egg, wheat toast w/o butter	1	2	2.7	200
2 Cholesterol-free eggs, wheat toast w/o butter	1	2	3.3	250
English muffin w/o butter	1	1-2	1.8	135
Cold Cereal w/2% milk Special K, Raisin Bran, Corn Flakes, Frosted Flakes	1	5	4.0	300
Hot Cereal				
Oatmeal	1 cup	2.5	2.0	150
Cream of Wheat	1 cup	1	2.4	180
with milk added		4.5	0.0	
Fruit Juice				
Chilled tomato	1	0	0.75	56.3
Grapefruit	1/2	0	1	75.0
Sliced fresh oranges	1	0	1	75.0
Applesauce	1	0	1	75.0
Sliced peaches	1	0	1	75.0
Stewed prunes	1	0	2	150.0
Sliced bananas	1	0	2	150.0
5 minute special orange juice, cereal, toast w/o butter, coffee	1	7.5	6.7-8	500-600
Super meal for kids Chilled juice, cereal, toast & hot chocolate	1	15	8.0	600
APPETIZERS:				
Farmers salad bowl w/o dressing	1	17	4.3	325
Tossed green salad	1	0	0.8	60
Gelatin salad	1	0	2.0	150
Spaghetti & meat sauce	1 cup	7.4	6.7	500

124

INTERSTATE HOLIDAY INN (continued)

ITEM	AMOUNT	FAT GRAMS	CALORIE PTS	CALORIES
HOUSE SPECIALTIES:				
Filet Mignon w/gelatin or tossed salad, mashed potatoes or baked potato & but	8 oz.	17	10.7	800
SEAFOOD:				
Broiled halibut w/lemon	8 oz.	7	3.0	225
SANDWICH SHOP:				
Club House w/o mayo (sandwich only)	1	14	5.9	440
French dip w/o fries	1	10.3	15.0	1125
Steak sand. w/o fries	1	14.2	6-6.7	450-500
DESSERTS:				
Sherbet	1	0	0.0	2

You'll enjoy the fine dining atmosphere, fresh and "home -prepared" foods at the sunny restaurant of the Interstate Holiday Inn Dining Room. Breakfasts are especially varied, yet the buffet, or ordering a dinner, sandwiches, or fresh salad will not be disappointing. Try them soon- a place for everyone.

MAX MAGRUDER'S

ITEM	AMOUNT	FAT GRAMS	CALORIE PTS	CALORIES
Cajun Chicken	Entree	13	6.3	472.5
Chicken Parmesan	Entree	17.5	8.5	637.5
Halibut	Entree	11	4.2	315
Chicken Gyro Sand.	1	21	7	525
Chicken Sandwich	1	13	5.5	412.5
Deli-Style Turkey Sand.	1	14.5	5.5	412.5
Hot Beef Sandwich	1	20	8.5	637.5
Nebraska Croissant	1	20.5	6	450
Cobb Salad	1	31.5	6	450
Dinner Salad	1	0	1	75
Junior Cobb Salad	1	15.75	3	225
Pink Salmon	8 oz.	10.1	4.5	337.5
Seafood Salad	1	2	2	150
Spinach Salad	1	33.5	5	375
Bacon Dressing	2 oz.	18	2.7	202.5
Creamy Italian Light	1 T.	4	0.5	37.5
French, Fat free	2T.	0	0.8	60
Mustard Dressing	2 oz.	19	3.3	247.5
Ranch Light	2 oz.	5.1	1	75
Cottage Cheese	1/2 cup	4.75	1.5	112.5
Soups:				
Bean with Ham	3/4 cup	2	2.5	187.5
Cheddar Cheese	3/4 cup	26	5.7	427.5
Cheddar & Cauliflower	3/4 cup	9	2.5	187.5
Chicken Noodle	3/4 cup	4	2.5	187.5
Chicken w/Wild Rice	3/4 cup	16	4.2	315
Chili	3/4 cup	18	5.3	397.5
Cream of Broccoli				
w/cheese	3/4 cup	16	3.5	262.5
Cream of Potato	3/4 cup	10	3.7	277.5
New England Clam				
Chowder	3/4 cup	26	5.7	427.5
Seafood Gumbo	1 cup	1.7	1.2	90

Shop - then - Stop - to choose from Max Magruder's variety of menu selections! You can choose from many salads, sandwiches, and entrees low in fat and low in calories. The staff at Max Magruder's will honor your requests for dressing on the side, or other fat and calorie saving changes that are healthy for your entire family!

NONNA'S

ITEM	AMOUNT	FAT GRAMS	CALORIE PTS	CALORIES
Cannelloni	1 serving	13	3.25	244
Spaghetti without meatballs	plate	5	5.2	390
Records Spaghetti	plate	21	8	600
Lean Lasagna	plate	7	3.5	263
Lasagna	plate	16.5	5.7	428
Lasagna	platter	25	8.7	653
Ravioli	platter	4	4.5	338
Chicken Breast w/Spaghetti	1 order	10	8	600
Meatballs	2	25	3.5	263
Homemade Olive Oil Dressing	2 T.	18	2	150
Italian Green Beans	1 serving	0	1	75
Strawberry Chantilly (omit whipped cream)	1	0	1	75

Nonna's has a well-written menu with different symbols to let you know about the different foods available. Apples on the menu indicate items prepared from natural ingredients. Hearts on the menu indicate items that are low in cholesterol. Nonna's only uses virgin olive oil in the food preparation. All the breads and pastas are made fat free. What you add to these products will determine the fat and calorie content of the final product.

Nutrition Matters gives Nonna's an A+ in the important area of providing their customers with the information needed to choose wisely.

PUMP AND PANTRY

ITEM	AMOUNT	FAT GRAMS	CALORIE PTS	CALORIES
HEART SMART SWEETS:				
Snackwells:				
Vanilla creme sandwich	2 cookies	2.5	1.5	110
Chocolate creme sand.	2 cookies	2.5	1.3	100
Devil's food cake	1 cookie	0	0.7	50
Doublefudge	1 cookie	0	0.7	50
Chocolate chip	6 cookies	0	0.8	60
Wheat crackers	5 crackers	0	0.8	60
Zesty cheese crackers	18 crackers	1	0.8	60
BW Fat Free Cobbler				
Raspberry	1 (2.25 oz.)	0	0.9	70
Apple	1 (2.25 oz.)	0	0.9	70
Grandma's sugar free wafers:				
Vanilla	1.48 oz.	7	2.7	200
Strawberry	1.48 oz.	7	2.7	200
3 Muskateers				
lower fat	1 (2.13 oz.)	8	3.5	260
Nabisco Phipps				
Original	1 oz.	4.5	1.6	120
BBQ	1 oz.	4	1.7	130
Sour Cream	1 oz.	4	1.7	130
Heartland Origionals				
Chicken fajita jerky	1 oz.	0	0.7	50
BBQ chicken breast	1 oz.	0.5	0.8	60
Dole Selcet Raisins	1 oz.	0	1.7	130
CHIPS & OTHER SNACKS:				
Sun Chips				
Harvest Cheddar	1 oz.	6	1.9	140
Original	1 oz.	6	1.9	140
French Onion	1 oz.	6	1.9	140
Rold Gold Pretzels	1 oz.	0	1.3	100
Vic's-lowfat popcorn				
White cheddar	2.5 cups	2.5	1.5	110
White popcorn	3.5 cups	1	1.5	110
MISC. ENTREES & SIDE DISHES:				
Oscar Mayer				
Nehring Farms	1 oz.	2	0.9	70
Lean Cuisine Teriyaki				
Stir Fry	9 oz.	5	3.5	260
Special K Cereal	1 cup	0	1.5	110

PUMP AND PANTRY (continued)

ITEM	AMOUNT	FAT GRAMS	CALORIE PTS	CALORIES
Misc. Entrees & Sides Dishes continued):				
Pepperidge Farms:				
Seasoned turkey gravy	2 oz.	1	0.4	30
Hearty beef gravy	2 oz.	1	0.3	25
Burritos	1 (5 oz.)	10	4.5	340
Billington Bakery				
fat free muffin	2 oz.	0	1.5	114.3
BEVERAGES:				
Very Fine juices				
Apple Quinchers	8 oz.	0	1.6	120
Grape	8 oz.	0	2.0	150
Fruit Punch	8 oz.	0	1.5	110
Orange	8 oz.	0	1.2	90
Orange juice 100%				
Roberts	8 oz.	0	1.6	120
Sunny Delight	8 oz.	0	1.5	110
Ultra Slim Fast, choc.	11 oz.	3	2.9	220
Cappuccino	6 oz.	3	1.2	90
Kay's Hot Chocolate	6 oz.	1	1.3	100
Yo Cream	1 oz.	0.7	0.3	23

Look who called! Bosselmans requested to get in the game of heart smart dining and wanted foods labeled and calculated for your benefit. Even in a hurry you can't miss the healthy selections available when you see the hot pink heart. Everything from snack foods, to quick grocery pick-ups can be found throughout the store at a low fat moderate calorie level, while a few "Your Advantage" foods continue to be popular for low fat, low salt or other benefits to you. Stop in at the Pump to prove you can eat healthy however fast the day's flying.....

RED LOBSTER

ITEM	AMOUNT	FAT GRAMS	CALORIE PTS	CALORIES
APPETIZERS:				
Shrimp Cocktail -				
(shrimp only)	6	0.5	0.7	50
Parmesan Zucchini	1	40	8.3	620
Stuffed Mushrooms	1	27	5.6	420
Lobster Stuffed				
Mushrooms	1	26	5.3	400
Fresh Fried Mushrooms	1	51	10.5	790
Chilled Shrimp in the				
Shell - shrimp 6 oz.	1	1.5	1.5	110
Chicken Fingers	1	18	5.2	390
Calamari	1	22	4.7	350
Crab & Shrimp Cakes	1	24	6.4	480
Mozzarella				
Cheesesticks	1	46	9.7	730
Lobster Quesadilla	1	47	10.1	760
Crab Add-on	1	1	0.8	60
Clam Chowder	6 oz.	5	1.7	130
Bayou Style Seafood	1			
Gumbo	6 oz.	4	1.6	120
Broccoli Cheese Soup	1 order	9	2.1	160
Shrimp Dinners:				
Shrimp Milano	1	65	15.9	1190
Fried Large Shrimp	12	27	6.7	500
Popcorn Shrimp	1	37	7.7	580
Shrimp Carbonara	1	76	17.2	1290
Shrimp Combo	1	23	5.1	380
Fish and Clam Dinners:				
Baked Atlantic Cod/				
Haddock	1	6	2.9	220
Catfish Santa Fe	1	9	4.5	340
Lemon Pepper Grilled				
Mahi Mahi	1	7	3.2	240
Clam Strips	1	39	9.6	720
Lobster and Crab Dinners:				
Live Maine Lobster,				
Steamed	1.25 lb.	1	2.1	160
Live Maine Lobster,				
Stuffed	2 lb.	10	5.7	430

RED LOBSTER (continued)

ITEM	AMOUNT	FAT GRAMS	CALORIE PTS	CALORIES
Lobster and Crab Dinners (continued):				
Broiled Rock Lobster				
Tail	1 tail	6	2.5	190
Snow Crab Legs	1	2	1.5	110
Crab Alfredo	1	66	15.6	1170
Seafood Combinations:				
Broiled Fisherman's				
Platter	1	23	8.0	600
Broiled Seafarer's	1	19	6.0	450
Neptune's Feast	1	62	16.1	1210
Lobster, Shrimp &				
Scallop Scampi	1	33	11.6	870
Fish & Shrimp Combo	1	35	9.7	730
Shrimp & Chicken	1	15	4.5	340
Shrimp Feast	1	24	6.3	470
Admiral's Feast	1	52	14.1	1060
Steaks and.......:				
New York Strip	1	34	7.5	560
Steak and Rock				
Lobster Tail	1	31	7.6	570
Steak & Fried Shrimp	1	46	10.4	780
Chicken Dinners:				
Grilled Chicken Breasts	1	7	3.1	230
Teriyaki Grilled Chicken				
Breast	1	7	3.2	240
Chicken Fresco	1	73	17.6	1320
Smothered Chicken	1	31	7.1	530
Salads:				
Shrimp Caesar Salad				
(no dressing)	1	11	3.2	240
Grilled Chicken Salad	1	10	4.3	320
Lunch:				
Catfish Santa Fe	1	6	2.4	180
Soup, Salad and				
Bread (no dressing)	1	18	5.7	430
Lobster, Shrimp &				
Scallop Scampi	1	16	5.7	430
Chicken Fingers	1	18	5.2	390

RED LOBSTER (continued)

ITEM	AMOUNT	FAT GRAMS	CALORIE PTS	CALORIES
Lunch (continued):				
Shrimp Milano	1	33	7.9	590
Popcorn Shrimp	1	24	5.1	380
Baked Flounder	1	7	2.5	190
Clam Strips	1	19	4.8	360
Fried Flounder	1	10	3.1	230
Crab Alfredo	1	33	7.9	590
Chicken Fresco	1	36	8.8	660
Fish Nuggets	1	14	4.3	320
Shrimp Carbonara	1	38	8.7	650
Seafood Broil	1	14	4.1	310
Sailor's Platter	1	12	3.3	250
Fried Shrimp	1	15	3.6	270
Lunch Sandwiches:				
Blackened Catfish Sandwich	1	9	4.5	340
Classic Fish Sand.	1	23	6.9	520
Broiled Fish Sand.	1	8	4.0	300
Grilled Chicken Sand.	1	7	3.9	290
Cajun Grilled Chicken Sandwich	1	14	4.9	370
Grilled Cheeseburger	1	34	7.7	580
Accompaniments:				
Baked Potato (flesh only)	8 oz.	0	1.7	130
Twice Baked Potato	1	23	5.7	430
French Fries	4 oz.	22	4.7	350
Rice Pilaf	4 oz.	2	2.4	180
Broccoli	3 oz.	0	0.3	25
Roasted Vegetables	6 oz. dinner	4	1.6	120
Roasted Vegetables	4 oz. lunch	3	1.1	80
Garden Salad (no dressing)	1	1	0.7	50
Caesar Salad (no dressing)	1	21	3.2	240
Cole Slaw	4 oz.	16	2.5	190
Applesauce	4 oz.	0	1.2	90
Garlic Cheese Bread	1 biscuit	8	1.9	140
Sauces/Dressings:				
Tarter Sauce	1 oz.	17	2.1	160

RED LOBSTER (continued)

ITEM	AMOUNT	FAT GRAMS	CALORIE PTS	CALORIES
Sauces and Dressings (continued):				
Cocktail Sauce	1 oz.	0	0.4	30
Sassy Sauce	1 oz.	6	1.1	80
Melted Butter	1 oz.	22	2.7	200
Marinara Sauce	1	4	0.7	50
Blue Cheese Dressing	1	18	2.3	170
Buttermilk Ranch Dressing	1	11	1.5	110
Dijon Honey Mustard	1	13	1.9	140
Fat Free Ranch Dressing	1	0	0.7	50
Lite Red Wine Vinaigrette Dressing	1	3	0.7	50
Caesar Dressing	1 oz.	18	2.3	170
Desserts:				
Cheesecake	5.5 oz.	41	7.1	530
Fudge Overboard	1	23	8.3	620
Ice Cream	4.5 oz.	7	1.9	140
Key Lime Pie	5 oz.	15	6.0	450
Carrot Cake	6.5 oz.	31	9.7	730
Sensational 7	1	41	9.7	790
Raspberry Cobbler	3 oz.	33	7.1	530
Child's:				
Fried Chicken Fingers	1	33	9.1	680
Popcorn Shrimp	1	35	8.7	650
Popcorn Shrimp & Cheesesticks	1	41	10.0	750
Fried Shrimp	1	33	8.7	650
Spaghetti with Cheesesticks	1	39	11.1	830
Grilled Chicken Tenders	1	24	7.7	580
Cheeseburger	1	56	13.9	1040
Hamburger	1	47	12.3	920
Fish:				
Catfish - Lunch	5 oz.	1.5	1.7	130
Catfish - Dinner	8 oz.	3	2.9	220
Atlantic Cod - Lunch	5 oz.	1	1.5	110
Atlantic Cod - Dinner	8 oz.	1.5	2.7	200
Flounder - Lunch	5 oz.	1.5	1.7	130

RED LOBSTER (continued)

ITEM	AMOUNT	FAT GRAMS	CALORIE PTS	CALORIES
Fish (continued):				
Flounder - Dinner	8 oz.	3	2.9	220
Grouper - Lunch	5 oz.	1.5	1.7	130
Grouper - Dinner	8 oz.	2.5	2.9	220
Haddock - Lunch	5 oz.	1	1.6	120
Haddock - Dinner	8 oz.	2	2.8	210
Halibut - Lunch	5 oz.	3.5	2.0	150
Halibut - Dinner	8 oz.	6	3.5	260
Mahi-Mahi - Lunch	5 oz.	1.5	1.7	130
Mahi-Mahi - Dinner	8 oz.	3	2.9	220
Perch - Lunch	5 oz.	1.5	1.7	130
Perch - Dinner	8 oz.	3	2.9	220
Pollock - Lunch	5 oz.	1.5	1.6	120
Pollock - Dinner	8 oz.	2.5	2.9	220
Red Rockfish - Lunch	5 oz.	2	1.7	130
Red Rockfish - Dinner	8 oz.	4	3.1	230
Red Snapper - Lunch	5 oz.	2	1.9	140
Red Snapper - Dinner	8 oz.	3	3.2	240
Atlantic Salmon-Lunch	5 oz.	9	2.7	200
Atlantic Salmon-Dinner	8 oz.	15	4.5	340
Sockeye Salmon - L	5 oz.	12	3.2	240
Sockeye Salmon - D	8 oz.	21	5.5	410
King Salmon - Lunch	5 oz.	15	3.3	250
King Salmon - Dinner	8 oz.	25	5.6	420
Sole - Lunch	5 oz.	1.5	1.7	130
Sole - Dinner	8 oz.	3	2.9	220
Swordfish - Lunch	5 oz.	6	2.3	170
Swordfish - Dinner	8 oz.	10	3.9	290
Lake Trout - Lunch	5 oz.	9	2.7	200
Lake Trout - Dinner	8 oz.	16	4.5	340
Walleye - Lunch	5 oz.	2	1.6	120
Walleye - Dinner	8 oz.	3	2.8	210
Yellow Lake Perch - L	5 oz.	1.5	1.7	130
Yellow Lake Perch - D	8 oz.	3	2.9	220
Seasonings:				
Broiled Fish - Lunch	1	4	0.5	35
Broiled Fish - Dinner	1	5	0.6	45
Grilled Fish - Lunch	1	3	0.3	25
Grilled Fish - Dinner	1	4	0.5	35
Lemon Pepper - Lunch	1	3	0.4	30

RED LOBSTER (continued)

ITEM	AMOUNT	FAT GRAMS	CALORIE PTS	CALORIES
Seasonings (continued):				
Lemon Pepper - Dinner	1	4	0.5	35
Santa Fe Style - Lunch	1	3	0.5	40
Santa Fe Style - Dinner	1	4	0.8	60
Blackened Fish-Lunch	1	4	0.7	50
Blackened Fish-Dinner	1	5	0.9	70

What a Menu....As Complete as you'll get with all foods on their new menu calculated for you . Even the smaller franchises offer all menu items that are evaluated for fat and calories by their national office. Seafood lovers here's your change in eating out, even in Nebraska for health and real food enjoyment all at one sitting.

RIVERSIDE GOLF CLUB

ITEM	AMOUNT	FAT GRAMS	CALORIE PTS	CALORIES
Weight Watchers Delight:				
*Tenderloin	4 oz.	13.5	6	450
*Chicken	4 oz.	4	5.7	425
*Halibut	6 oz.	5	5.9	440
*Served with vegetables & fruit				
Orange Roughy Dinner				
w/veg.,tossed salad				
& baked potato				
(w/o butter or dressing)	1 dinner	16.4	8.0	600
w/o baked potato	1 dinner	16.4	5.3	400
Chicken Breast Sand.				
(w/o mayonnaise)	1 sandwich	8.2	5.5	415
Sliced Turkey Sand.				
(w/o mayonnaise)				
6 oz. fruit	1	4.9	4.9	370
Caesar Salad with				
chicken breast				
(w/o dressing)				
2/6 oz. fruit	1	6.3	4.1	310
The Sandbagger				
Tomato slices, cottage				
cheese, fruit				
*with chicken	1	9	5.1	383
*with halibut	1	7.1	5.6	420
Slice:				
*Meat, 2 slices white				
bread, 2 slices wheat				
bread, 2 slices rye				
bread, lettuce,				
tomatoes, cheese				
*w/roast beef	1	19.2	6.4	477
*w/turkey	1	12.5	5.9	443
*w/lean ham	1	17.3	5.7	428

When you want health and fine dining,members of Riverside have the advantage. Ann Ottman and staff have the ability to meet your health needs with quality foods and the finest preparation. Ask your waitress for suggestions on fish, poultry, and side dish entrees prepared low in fat and moderate in sodium. Steamed vegetables and fruit mixtures are always available to accompany your entree of choice.

SAM'S CLUB

ITEM	AMOUNT	FAT GRAMS	CALORIE PTS	CALORIES
MEATS:				
Butterball				
smoked turkey breast	1 slice	1	0.4	30
Mr. Turkey				
smoked turkey breast	1 slice	0.5	0.4	30
Hudson				
chicken breast portion	6 oz.	14	3.3	247.5
chicken breast				
(boneless, skinless)	4 tenders	0.5	1.4	105
chicken Mesquite				
breast fillets	1 portion	2.5	1.2	90
chicken glazed				
breast fillets	1 portion	3.5	1.3	97.5
chicken honey				
mustard	1 portion	5	1.6	120
Tyson dice chicken				
meat	2/3 cup	4	1.7	127.5
Dak Premuim Ham	2 slices	2	0.8	60
Hudson				
99% fat free chicken				
fajita	1 fajita	1	2.0	150
stir-fry beef	1 cup	2	2.4	180
stir-fry chicken	1 cup	4	2.1	157.5
stir-fry shrimp	1 cup	1	1.3	97.5
stir-fry vegetables	3/4 cup	0	0.5	37.5
Shanghai stir-fry				
shrimp & vegetables	1 3/4 cup	1	1.2	90
Tyson				
Oriental beef w/veg	1 cup	3	2.3	172.5
Chicken breast & fried rice	1 cup	0	2.4	180
Skinless chicken				
breast & stir-fry	1 cup	0	1.6	120
Michael Angelos				
chicken lasagna	1 cup	6	3.3	247.5
w/meat sauce	1 cup	14	4.4	330
Overbrook chicken &				
pasta w/veg.	1 cup	2.5	2.4	180
Healthy Choice				
breast of turkey	10.5 oz.	3	3.7	277.5
salisbury steak	11 oz.	6	3.5	262.5
traditional beef tips	11.25 oz.	5	3.5	262.5
pepper fish	10.7 oz.	5	3.9	292.5
pasta shells marinara	12 oz.	4	4.9	367.5

SAM'S CLUB (continued)

ITEM	AMOUNT	FAT GRAMS	CALORIE PTS	CALORIES
MEATS (continued):				
Healthy Choice (continued)				
roast turkey	10 oz.	4	3.3	247.5
Mesquite chicken barbecue	10.5 oz.	2	4.3	322.5
sesame chicken shanghai	12 oz.	5	4.1	307.5
Lean Cuisine				
sweet & chicken	1/2 cup	2.5	1.5	112.5
glazed chicken	1 pkg.	6	3.2	240
chicken & veg.	1 pkg.	5	3.2	240
macaroni & cheese	1 cup	14	4.7	352.5
Pierre chicken breast				
sandwich	1 sandwich	8	3.5	262.5
Oceans Original				
orange roughy	4 oz.	8	1.9	142.5
ocean perch	4 oz.	1	1.3	97.5
flounder	4 oz.	1.5	1.3	97.5
cod fillets	4 oz.	0.5	1.2	90
Butterball fat free turkey				
breast. variety	4 slices	0	0.7	52.5
Alpine Lace sliced cheese	1 slice	0	0.3	22.5
American Fitness				
Classic energy bar	1 bar	2	2.8	210
Tahitian Tropics fruit bar	1 bar	0	2.4	180
Healthy Valley				
choc. breakfast bar	1 bar	0	1.5	112.5
straw. breakfast bar	1 bar	0	1.9	142,5
fruit & fitness bar	1 bar	0	1.4	105
straw. cookie	1 cookie	0	1.1	82.5
Nature Valley lowfat				
granola bar	2 bars	3	2.1	157.5
Newton's fat free				
variety pak	1 cookie	0	1.0	75
Snackwell's				
cream sandwich	2 cookies	2.5	1.4	105
devils food	1 cookie	0	0.7	52.5
variety pak -cracked pepper	7 crackers	0	0.8	60
wheat	5 crackers	0	0.8	60
classic golden	10 cracker	1	0.8	60

SAM'S CLUB (continued)

ITEM	AMOUNT	FAT GRAMS	CALORIE PTS	CALORIES
Keebler low fat graham crackers	8 crackers	1.5	1.5	112.5
Keebler fudge strips	3 strips	4.5	1.7	127.5
Townhouse reduced fat crackers	6 crackers	2	0.9	67.5
Kellogg's lowfat granola with raisins	2/3 cup	3	2.8	210
Healthy Valley fat free potato snack	1 1/2 cup	0	1.3	97.5
Super soft pretzels	1	0	2.2	165
Bloomfield brownies	2 bars	0	1.7	127.5
Tahitian Tropics fruit bar	1 bar	2	2.4	180
Krusteaz apple muffins	1 muffin	0	1.7	127.5
blueberry muffin	1 muffin	0	1.7	127.5
Rold Gold fat free pretzels	1 oz.	0	1.5	112.5
Tostitos, baked	1 oz.	0	1.4	105
Louise's fat free chips	1 oz.	0	1.3	97.5
Hershey's reduced fat baking chips	1 t.	3.5	0.8	60
Carnation sugar free choc. mix	1 env.	0	0.7	52.5
Log Cabin "lite" reduced calorie syrup	1/4 cup	0	1.3	97.5
Kraft fat free Ranch	2 T.	0	0.7	52.5
Italian	2 T.	0	0.7	52.5
Honey Dijon	2 T.	0	0.7	52.5
Marzetti fat free Ceasar dressing	2 T.	0	0.3	22.5
Red wine dressing	2 T.	0	0.5	37.5
Italian dressing	2 T.	0	0.2	15
Hormel veg. chili w/ beans (canned)	1 cup	0	2.7	202.5
Yoplait double fruit fat free bar	1 bar	0	0.6	45

SAM'S CLUB (continued)

ITEM	AMOUNT	FAT GRAMS	CALORIE PTS	CALORIES
Edy's fat free ice cream				
vanilla	1/2 cup	0	1.2	90
chocolate	1/2 cup	0	1.2	90
strawberry	1/2 cup	0	1.2	90
raspberry	1/2 cup	0	1.1	82.5
choc. brownie chunk	1/2 cup	0	1.6	12
caramel praline crun.	1/2 cup	0	1.5	112.5
black cherry vanilla	1/2 cup	0	1.3	97.5
heath toffee crunch	1/2 cup	0	1.6	120

Sam's has what you need. If you haven't joined Sam's for any other reason, some of the great buys on lean meats would be one reason to open a membership. You'll see this list of products continues to grow, as new products come on the market. The foods will change, yet a large selection of portioned foods and basic lean foods will be there for your menu plan-always available plus the dollar savings is obvious. Check our Sam's soon.....

TAYLOR'S STEAK HOUSE AND CATERING

ITEM	AMOUNT	FAT GRAMS	CALORIE PTS	CALORIES
FISH:				
Swordfish	8 oz.	22.5	5.3	397.5
Salmon	8 oz.	2	2.2	165
Halibut	8 oz.	11	5.3	397.5
Scallops	8 oz.	1.4	2.4	180
Broiled Trout	8 oz.	8	3.7	277.5
Shrimp Cocktail:				
Shrimp	4 oz.	2	1.5	112.5
Sauce	1/4 cup	0	1	75
Salmon w/dill sauce	8 oz.	3.8	2.7	202.5
CHICKEN:				
Br. Chicken Breast	6 oz.	4	2.6	195
Rice	4 oz.	0	1	75
Mozzarella Chicken Breast w/mozz. cheese and sauce	6 oz.	24.2	7.2	540
BEEF:				
Top Sirloin Steak	8 oz.	15.5	5.8	435
Super Lean Hamburger	5 oz.	18	4	302
SALAD:				
Greek Salad	1 serving	14.5	5	375
Vinaigrette Dressing	3.25 oz.	40	5.2	390
Chicken Salad	1 serving	3	3.1	232.5
Hidden Valley Dressing	2 oz.	1.5	0.5	37.5
SANDWICHES:				
Chicken Sandwich	1 sandwich	11	6	450
Tuna Melt	1 sandwich	23.8	6.8	510
SOUPS:				
Tomato Cabbage	8 oz.	0	0.9	67.5
Minestrone	8 oz.	0.3	2.2	165
PIE:				
Sugar Free Apple Pie 1 slice	1/6 pie	6.6	3	225

Pam, Tom, and Staff at Taylor's have dedicated themselves to quality foods- from the fresh lean meats to all the other top of the line ingredients for a meal that is quality for You! The staff works hard to keep the customer's health as well as their appetites satisfied.

U-SAVE

At U-Save Grocery there are thousands of food items to fit into a healthy food plan. We can only feature a few of those, but feel this page should inform you of brand names that may add healthy additions to a flexible food plan.

Bakery: Tim and his staff make many wonderful breads truly from "scratch". You may appreciate the bagels, whole grain breads, and fat free brownies for meals and snacks. (Try a fresh Petrofsky's Bagel - 270 calories and 3 grams of fat)

Bakery Items: Hersheys" reduced fat chocolate chips, Krusteaz fat free muffins, Betty Crocker light brownies are just a few of the calorie and fat savers in this aisle. Packaged items: Mission Fat Free Tortillas, Millspring Bagels, Sweet Reward Brownie Mixes, Fat Free Sugar Cookies: Auburn Farm Health Valley. Frozen Breads: Rhodes Fat Free Rolls, Whole Wheatrolls, White Rolls,

Beverages: Sugar Free General Foods Flavored Coffees, Crystal Light Drinks, Many brands instant decaf coffees, and decaf teas, sugar free pops ,

Butter Flavorings: Molly McButter, Butter Buds, I can't believe its not Butter, Fleischmans Corn and Rice Cakes: Quaker, Hain, and Act Two

Candy: Brach's Fat Free Jels, Hershey's Sweet Escapes, Diet Farley's Candy, Sorbee , Estee, and Vivil sugar free candies, Delicious candy.

Cheeses: Healthy Favorites Fat Free, Krafts fat free and reduced, l/3 less

Dairy: Our Family and Cool Whip Light topping, Kraft and Meadow Gold Fat Free Dips, Daisy and Meadow Gold Fat Free Sour Cream, Viva Light Sour Cream, HealthWise Milk, Viva Fortified Skim and l%, Viva Nonfat Cottage Cheese, Scramblers and Egg Beaters Egg Substitutes, Healthy Choice, Fairmont, Lite/ Gillette, Eskimo Pie, Lite Time Gillette ice creams. Fat Free Sugar free Yogurts: Lite 85, Weight Watchers 90.

Deli: Featuring lean meats, vegetable and pasta salads. Many lean meats from Oscar Mayer, Louis Rich, and other quality brand names with a variety of foods made from polyunsaturated oils. We feature personal touch catering for any event that comes your way. This new department will save you time, calories and fat while making meals easy to put on the table.

Entrees: Weight Watchers, Lean Cuisine, Budget Gourmet Light, Healthy Choice, Green Giant, Swanson come in a variety of entrees and complete dinners low in fat and calories.

U-SAVE (continued)

Meats: Packaged meats-Light and Lean Hormel, Deli Select, Oscar Mayer Light, Louis Rich, Jimmy Dean Tastefully Done, Lunchables, Light, Lunchables, Imitation Crab, John Morrell 50% less fat Franks, Extra Lean Swift Ground Beef

Pastas: <u>Frozen</u>: Rosetto Ravioli, Pasta Cafe Tortellinis, Fat Free Reame Noodles, and Aunt Vi Fat Free and Low Fat Noodles.

Potatoes: Lyndon Farms, Our Family, Vita Bite, Mr. Dells, Ore Ida: varying amount of fat added so read labels carefully.

Salad Dressings: Weight Watchers, Estee, Low calorie, Kraft Fat Free, Hidden Valley Fat Free and Light, Western Fat Free, Seven Seas' Free, Dorothy Lynch Reduced Calorie

Soups: Campbells' Healthy Request, Healthy Choice, Knorr's, Swanson, Weight Watchers, Healthy Recipe.

Syrups: Light Knotts, reduced sugar, Sugar Free Vermont, Cary's Sugar Free.

VILLAGE INN

ITEM	AMOUNT	FAT GRAMS	CALORIE PTS	CALORIES
BREAKFAST HEART SMART FOODS:				
Cinnamon Raisin Toast	1 order	15.5	10.7	802.5
Low Cholesterol Fruit & Nut Pancake	1 order	19	12.5	937.5
Fresh Veg. Omelet	1 order	18.33	9.5	712.5
Chicken & Veggie Omelet	1 order	18.75	9.5	712.5
Dry Cereals (see Cereal)				
2% Milk	1 cup	5	1.5	112.5
Pancakes (short stack)	1 order	11.25	4.5	337.5
Waffle	1 only	17.5	6	450
LUNCH AND DINNER ITEMS (No side dishes included):				
Turkey Garden Vegetable Grill	1 order	17.75	5	375
Grilled Chicken Sand. w/Tomato	1 order	16	7	525
Grilled Chicken Sand. Plain	1 order	8	5.7	427.5
Light Grilled Fish	1 order	8	2.5	187.5
French Dip Sand. w/mashed potatoes	1 order	16	6.2	465
Lighter Side Grilled Chicken Breast w/ egg & 1/2 cup cottage cheese	1 order	22	4.25	318.75
Mini Chef Salad	1 order	17	4	300
Light French Dressing	1 T.	3	0.5	37.5

Village Inn isn't just for breakfasts anymore... Anytime of the day you'll want to try an entree from a menu full of variety, low fat, delicious foods. There is no reason to leave your "heart healthy" plan at home when you have eggbeaters, toasted breads, grilled sandwiches and other lean choices. All of the Heart Smart breakfast items are less than 30% fat. Remember Village Inn all times of the day, when you want healthful and satisfying food.

YEN CHING

ITEM	AMOUNT	FAT GRAMS	CALORIE PTS	CALORIES
SPECIALTIES:				
Hunan Shrimp	1 dinner	8.2	4.8	361
	1 lunch	5.8	3.2	241
Scallops w/Hunan	1 dinner	5.2	3.6	271
Sauce	1 lunch	4.5	2.4	181
Shrimp /Black Bean	1 dinner	8.9	4.8	361
Sauce	1 lunch	6.2	3.2	241
Squid w/Szechuan	1 dinner	8	4.3	324
Sauce	1 lunch	5.7	2.9	219
Summer Special	1 dinner	14.9	5.6	421
	1 lunch	10.2	3.7	279
HOUSE SPECIALTIES:				
Chicken w/Black	1 dinner	10.9	4.8	361
Bean Sauce	1 lunch	7.6	3.2	241
Garden Scallops	1 dinner	7	3.9	290
	1 lunch	5	2.6	196
Ton Ting Shrimp	1 dinner	7.5	4.6	346
	1 lunch	5.3	3.1	234
SEAFOOD:				
Empress Scallops	1 dinner	6.2	4.4	330
	1 lunch	4.5	2.9	219
Shrimp w/Garlic Sauce	1 dinner	8.9	4.8	360
	1 lunch	6.3	3.2	241
Shrimp w/Snow Peas	1 dinner	8.6	5.2	387
	1 lunch	6.1	3.4	256
Sizzling Happy Family	1 dinner	15	9.9	744
	1 lunch	10.3	6.6	496
Three Treasures of	1 dinner	7.8	3.6	270
the Sea	1 lunch	5.5	2.4	181
BEEF:				
Beef w/Fresh Broccoli	1 dinner	17.2	5.6	421
	1 lunch	11.8	3.7	279
Beef w/Snow Peas	1 dinner	17.2	5.9	444
	1 lunch	11.8	3.9	294
Pepper Steak	1 dinner	17.2	5.9	444
	1 lunch	11.8	3.9	294

YEN CHING (continued)

ITEM	AMOUNT	FAT GRAMS	CALORIE PTS	CALORIES
FOWL:				
Almond Chicken	1 dinner	25.3	8.3	624
	1 lunch	17.2	4.9	369
Chicken w/Garlic	1 dinner	10.9	6.0	450
Sauce	1 lunch	7.6	3.4	252
Kung Pao Chicken	1 dinner	23.9	7.5	564
	1 lunch	16.2	5.0	376
Mandarin Chicken	1 dinner	10.9	5.3	399
	1 lunch	7.6	3.3	249
Phoenix & Dragon	1 dinner	9	4.9	365
	1 lunch	6.5	3.4	252
Snow White Chicken	1 dinner	10.9	5.1	381
	1 lunch	7.6	4.4	333
PORK:				
Hunan Pork:	1 dinner	22.4	6.9	518
	1 lunch	15.2	4.6	346
VEGETABLES:				
Bean Curd w/Fresh	1 dinner	5	4.2	312
Vegetables	1 lunch	3.7	2.8	211
Broccoli & Mushrooms	1 dinner	4.5	3.4	253
w/Oyster Sauce	1 lunch	3.3	1.5	113
Empress Vegetable	1 dinner	6.2	2.6	196
Deluxe Dinner	1 lunch	4.5	1.9	141
Fresh Mushrooms	1 dinner	6.6	4.8	361
w/Bean Curd	1 lunch	4.7	2.5	189
Snow Pea Delight	1 dinner	3.8	2.6	196
	1 lunch	2.8	1.7	131
Three Ingredient	1 dinner	6.7	4.3	325
Vegetables	1 lunch	4.8	2.2	166

Your future will look good if you start eating at Yen Ching on 2nd Street or South Locust. Mein and her staff have been health conscious for years! Their use of small amounts of sesame oil is obvious when you look at the fat grams listed above. They also stir-fry without MSG. Your waiter will be attentive to your requests, for your favorite Chinese food to be guilt free. Anyone wanting a meat free dish Yen Ching has many to choose from.

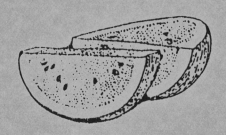

DINING OUT FOR GOOD HEALTH

  Methodist Hospital and many area restaurants along with a number of corporate cafeterias have joined together to provide the "A Fare of the Heart" program to make your food selections nutritious, tasty and healthful, even when dining out. "A'fare of the Heart" is a special dietary program with selected menus of heart-wise appetizers, entrees, side dishes, beverages and even desserts. These selected items are low in cholesterol, fat and sodium.

OMAHA A'FARE OF THE HEART
Lincoln & Omaha Restaurants

ITEM	AMOUNT	FAT GRAMS	CALORIE PTS	CALORIES
ANGELO'S PIZZA & PASTA:				
PIZZA PER SLICE				
Chicken, Broccoli,Tomato-				
Thin		4	2.2	163
Pan		4	2.9	217
Heartland Healthy-				
Thin		6	2.4	178
Pan		6	3.1	232
Shrimp, Onion, Green Pepper-				
Thin		3		
Pan		3	2.7	206
Hawaiian Pizza-				
Thin		4	2.2	166
Pan		4	2.9	220
Veggie Pizza-				
Thin		4	2.0	149
Pan		4	2.7	203
BBQ Chicken-				
Thin		4	2.3	176
Pan		4	3.1	230
Garden Salad		2	1.0	76
Dinner Salad		0	0.2	17
Pasta w/Marinara				
Sauce-Ala Carte		3	2.9	216
Dinner		5	4.5	341
Pasta w/Meat				
Sauce-Ala Carte		9	3.9	294
Dinner		13	6.1	456
Pasta w/Pesto-				
Ala Carte		5	2.6	197
Dinner		9	4.5	335
Linguine w/ Napoli				
Vegetables-Ala Carte		7	3.3	248
Dinner		11	5.2	388
Mostacioli Mancini				
Pomodoro-Ala Carte		3	3.2	237
Dinner		4	4.9	371
Linguine w/Chicken				
Pesto-Ala Carte		8	4.7	349
Dinner		13	7.0	523

OMAHA A'FARE OF THE HEART
Lincoln & Omaha Restaurants (continued)

ITEM	AMOUNT	FAT GRAMS	CALORIE PTS	CALORIES
Angelo's Pizza & Pasta (continued):				
Linguine w/Shrimp				
Pesto-Ala Carte		5	3.4	257
Dinner		10	5.5	413
Baked Spaghetti				
Supremo-Ala Carte		13	5.0	372
Dinner		19	7.7	581
Chicken Parmeasan-				
Ala Carte		9	4.0	303
Dinner		11	6.5	489
Orange Sherbet		3	2.7	202
BAKER'S:				
Breakfast #1		4	4.9	364
Breakfast #2		2	5.1	379
Breakfast #3		5	4.2	313
Entree #1		3	3.0	223
Entree #2				
Fruit &Hard Roll w/FF Chicken				
&Macaroni Salad		6	5.8	433
w/FF Tuna & Macaroni Salad		3	5.3	395
w/FF Tuna & Potato Salad		3	5.1	380
w/FF Chicken & Potato Salad		6	5.6	418
Entree #3				
w/ Fresh Fruit & FF Tuna Salad		1	2.3	174
w/FF Chicken Salad		4	2.8	211
Entree #4				
w/FF Macaroni Salad		11	6.4	480
w/FF Potato Salad		11	6.2	465
Dessert #1		1	1.7	130
Dessert #2		0	1.6	120

ITEM	AMOUNT	FAT GRAMS	CALORIE PTS	CALORIES
FERNANDO'S:				
Chicken Taco		8	3.2	238
Deluxe Taco		12	4.8	361
Chicken Enchilada		10	4.4	327
Bean Burrito		10	6.5	489
Bean Tostada		7	4.2	318
Seafood Enchilada		12	4.9	369
Fajita Salad		12	5.3	401
Grilled Chicken Sandwich				
with Rice and Salad		12	7.2	539
Cool Lime Pie		7	4.2	316
GAETA'S RESTAURANT:				
Minestrone Soup-Cup		0	0.6	44
Bowl		0	0.8	57
Chef's Creation		10	4.8	360
Grilled Chicken Filet		4	4.8	363
French Dip		14	6.4	478
Halibut Steak		8	3.8	284
Lemon Baked Cod		10	3.8	282
1/2 Lemon Baked Cod		5	1.9	141
Chicken Breast American		4	2.3	171
Spaghetti & Meat Sauce				
& Garlic Toast		16	7.2	543
SIDE DISHES:				
Spaghetti		3	1.6	119
Cottage Cheese		2	0.9	68
Fruit		0	0.6	45
Salad		0	0.1	5
Baked Potato		0	2.2	165
Vegetable		0	0.2	18

OMAHA A'FARE OF THE HEART
Lincoln & Omaha Restaurants (continued)

ITEM	AMOUNT	FAT GRAMS	CALORIE PTS	CALORIES
GARDEN CAFE:				
Heart Fruit Plate				
w/Lowfat Muffin		2	6.8	508
w/Bran Muffin		12	7.2	538
Heart French Toast				
w/Applesauce		3	4.3	324
w/Low Cal Syrup		3	4.9	368
Heart Omelette				
w/Fruit		2	3.0	227
w/Lowfat Muffin		2	5.0	375
w/Bran Muffin		12	5.4	405
Heart Chicken Stirfry				
w/Lowfat Muffin		5	5.9	445
w/Bran Muffin		14	6.3	475
w/Dinner Roll		6	3.7	280
Heart Italian Chicken				
w/Rice		6	6.3	473
Polynesian Chicken				
w/Rice		3	6.2	464
Heart Halibut Dinner				
w/Rice		6	5.5	410
Heart Potato Casserole				
w/Lowfat Muffin		12	9.4	702
w/Bran Muffin		21	9.8	732
w/Dinner Roll		13	7.2	538
Heart Jacket Potato				
w/Fruit		12	5.8	433
Heart Salad w/Dole Whip				
& Lowfat Muffin		8	6.6	493
& Bran Muffin		17	7.0	523
& Dinner Roll		10	4.4	328
Heart Spinach Salad				
w/Lowfat Muffin		5	5.4	408
w/ Bran Muffin		14	5.8	438
w/ Dinner Roll		7	3.3	244
Heart Chef Salad				
w/Lowfat Muffin		10	7.3	551
w/Bran Muffin		19	7.7	581
w/Dinner Roll		12	5.1	386
Heart French Dip				
w/Fruit		7	4.5	335

OMAHA A'FARE OF THE HEART
Lincoln & Omaha Restaurants (continued)

ITEM	AMOUNT	FAT GRAMS	CALORIE PTS	CALORIES
Garden Cafe (continued):				
Heart Chicken Sandwich				
w/Fruit		16	6.8	512
Heart Melt				
w/Fruit		10	4.4	330
GORAT'S STEAK HOUSE:				
Petit Filet Mignon w/Cottage				
Cheese, Vegetable, &				
Baked Potato		15	6.5	490
w/Salad, Vegetable, &				
Baked Potato		14	5.1	380
Weight Watcher Sirloin w/				
Cottage Cheese,				
Vegetable & Baked Potato		11	6.1	454
w/Salad, Vegetable, &				
Baked Potato		9	4.6	344
Halibut Steak w/ Cottage				
Cheese, Vegetable, &				
Baked Potato		6	5.5	410
w/Salad, Vegetable, &				
Baked Potato		4	4.0	300
Orange Roughy w/ Cottage				
Cheese, Vegetable,				
& Baked Potato		11	5.1	386
w/Salad, Vegetable, &				
Baked Potato		9	3.5	266
Skinless Chicken Breast w/				
Cottage Cheese, Vegetable,				
& Baked Potato		4	5.1	380
w/Salad, Vegetable,				
& Baked Potato		2	3.5	260
Sherbet		2	1.8	135
Frozen Yogurt		2	1.9	140

151

OMAHA A'FARE OF THE HEART
Lincoln & Omaha Restaurants (continued)

ITEM	AMOUNT	FAT GRAMS	CALORIE PTS	CALORIES
GREAT AMERICAN DINER:				
Garden Platter		1	0.8	61
Chicken Breast Sandwich w/Melon		10	6.9	519
Salmon Catch w/rice, vegetable melon, salad, & roll		20	8.7	651
Chicken Stir Fry w/rice, salad, & dinner roll		6	6.7	536
Chicken Salad		3	3.2	242
Spinach Salad		4	1.7	129
Health Salad		5	2.1	161
Dinner Salad		3	1.2	87
Sherbet		3	2.7	203
Frozen Yogurt		5	1.8	135
1/2 Cantaloupe w/Frozen Yogurt		5	3.1	229
Frozen Yogurt w/Low Fat Chocolate Topping		5	3.4	255
Lite & Fluffy Omelette		2	3.0	226
Hot cereal w/berries & toast		3	2.4	183
Hot cereal w/ bananas & toast		3	3.7	278
Cold cereal w/berries & toast		2	2.7	205
Cold cereal w/bananas & toast		2	4.0	300
Lite French Toast w/low-cal syrup		2	4.9	368
Bagel w/cream cheese & fruit		5	6.4	479
Bran muffin w/juice		10	5.5	414
Bran Muffin w/fruit		11	5.8	435
JACK & MARY'S:				
Fresh Veggie Combo w/Dip		2	1.7	124
Citrus Chicken Salad w/Citrus Muffin & Vinaigrette		11	8.8	663
Barbecued Chicken Salad w/ Barbecue Vinaigrette		14	5.6	421

OMAHA A'FARE OF THE HEART
Lincoln & Omaha Restaurants (continued)

ITEM	AMOUNT	FAT GRAMS	CALORIE PTS	CALORIES
Jack & Mary's (continued):				
Grilled Chicken w/Mashed				
Potatoes & Salad		4	3.4	256
w/Mashed Potatoes &				
Cottage Cheese		7	4.7	353
w/Vegetable & Cottage Cheese		4	3.9	291
w/Vegetable & Salad		2	2.6	194
Charbroiled Halibut w/Mashed				
Potatoes & Salad		6	3.9	291
w/Mashed Potatoes & Cottage				
Cheese		8	5.2	388
w/Vegetable & Cottage Cheese		6	4.3	326
w/Vegetable & Salad		4	3.1	229
Charbroiled Salmon w/				
Vegetable & Salad		9	3.6	269
w/Vegetable & Cottage Cheese		11	4.6	357
JOHNNY'S CAFE:				
French Onion Soup		1	0.5	36
Salmon Seafood Salad		6	2.5	187
Tuna Seafood Salad		2	2.2	166
Johnny's House Salad		0	0.2	14
Fruit Jello Salad		0	1.2	92
Luncheon Salad		0	0.2	16
Cottage Cheese Spread per				
Tablespoon		0.2	0.2	13
Johnny's Luncheon Steak w/				
Mashed Potatoes, Salad, &				
Dinner Roll		11	5.1	383
w/Mashed Potatoes, Applesauce				
& Dinner Roll		11	4.5	341
From the Wok:				
Shrimp		6	4.0	301
Chicken Breast		6	4.0	300
Beef		10	5.0	372
Vegetarian		5	3.2	238

OMAHA A'FARE OF THE HEART
Lincoln & Omaha Restaurants (continued)

ITEM	AMOUNT	FAT GRAMS	CALORIE PTS	CALORIES
Johnny's Cafe (continued):				
Golden Brown Halibut Steak w/Mashed Potatoes, Salad, & Dinner Roll		7	5.4	404
w/Mashed Potatoes, Applesauce & Dinner Roll		7	6.0	447
Broiled Orange Roughy w/ Mashed Potatoes, Salad, & Dinner Roll		13	5.3	396
w/Mashed Potatoes, Applesauce & Dinner Roll		13	5.8	438
Individual Northern Catfish w/ Mashed Potatoes, Salad, & Dinner Roll		7	4.7	352
w/Mashed Potatoes, Applesauce & Dinner Roll		7	5.3	395
Broiled Ginger Chicken Breast w/ Mashed Potatoes, Salad, & Dinner Roll		5	5.0	373
w/Mashed Potatoes, Applesauce & Dinner Roll		5	5.5	416
Sherbert		2		135
Johnny's Special Salad Bowl		2		62
Wedge of Lettuce Salad		0	0.1	11
Shrimp Salad		2	1.6	122
Petite Filet w/Baked Potato, Salad, Cottage Cheese, & Roll		18	9.3	700
Broiled Orange Roughy w/ Baked Potato, Salad, Cottage Cheese, & Roll		15	7.8	587
Northwest Halibut w/Baked Potato, Salad, Cottage Cheese, & Roll		10	7.6	567
Broiled Ginger Chicken Breast w/ Baked Potato, Salad, Cottage Cheese, & Roll		5	6.7	505

ITEM	AMOUNT	FAT GRAMS	CALORIE PTS	CALORIES

JONESY'S DINNER DEN:

ITEM	AMOUNT	FAT GRAMS	CALORIE PTS	CALORIES
Mini Fresh Fruit Plate		0	1.0	75
Raw Vegetable Relish Tray		0	0.3	21
3 Slices Fresh Tomato w/Basil &Cottage Cheese		1	0.7	49
Summer Chicken Salad w/Muffin		16	7.1	535
w/Dinner Roll		10	4.8	363
Chef Salad w/Whole Wheat Roll		10	4.5	335
Custer Salad		3	3.1	236
Club Steak w/Sliced Tomato, Salad, & 1/2 Baked Potato		14	6.3	473
Halibut Steak w/Salad, Wild Rice & Vegetable		6	5.5	411
Grilled Chicken Breast w/Cottage Cheese Stuffed Tomato & Fruit		8	5.4	402
Grilled Chicken over Rice w/ Salad & Roll		4	4.5	341
Grilled Quail w/ Salad & Rice		8	4.5	339
Ice Cream Alternative Dessert		0	1.1	80
Mini Fresh Fruit Plate		0	1.0	75
Pound Cake Topped w/ Red Raspberries & Frozen Dessert		0	1.5	110

JULIO'S:

ITEM	AMOUNT	FAT GRAMS	CALORIE PTS	CALORIES
Tex-Mex Chili Cup w/1 Tortilla		6	2.3	174
Julio's Health Salad		3	1.3	96
Taco Chic Riced		16	6.3	471
Burrito Bopper w/Rice		15	6.4	479
Fro-Yo-Yum		4	1.5	112

OMAHA A'FARE OF THE HEART
Lincoln & Omaha Restaurants (continued)

ITEM	AMOUNT	FAT GRAMS	CALORIE PTS	CALORIES
METHODIST HOSTPITAL:				
Turkey Hero		4	3.7	275
Roast Beef Hero		7	4.6	345
Dinner Salad		0	0.3	25
Garden Salad		0	0.5	35
Turkey Lite		2	2.2	165
Beefeater Lite		5	2.9	215
M'S PUB:				
Seafood Ceviche		9	3.5	264
M's House Salad w/lowfat dill dressing		3	2.7	203
Spinach Salad w/lowfat dill dressing		10	4.2	317
Pork Tenderloin Salad w/Vinaigrette		8	4.9	365
Salmon Salad w/Vinaigrette		12	7.0	527
Three Bird Salad w/Vinaigrette		21	8.9	667
Chicken Tenderloin Salad w/Vinaigrette		7	4.9	364
Turkey Burger w/Non-fat Mayo		14	7.2	537
Fish Burger w/Non-fat Tartar Sauce		11	6.0	450
Chicken Burger w/Non-fat Mayo		14	6.7	502
Carrot Dog		4	5.7	429
Indian Chicken w/Rice & Spicy Yogurt Sauce		5	5.5	409
Floyd's Skinny Plate w/Chicken		5	3.8	285
w/Salmon		9	3.8	285
THE MARKET BASKET:				
Heart Healthy Omelette w/Toast		12	5.0	372
Good Morning Pancakes		7	3.4	255
Heart Healthy Deli Delight w/Fruit		13	7.7	581
Heart Healthy California w/Fruit		15	6.9	516
Southwestern Grilled Chicken Salad w/Roll		10	6.5	484
Garden Salad w/Roll		3	2.7	200
Fresh Fruits of the Season w/Roll		4	4.8	361
Steamed Vegetables w/Roll		3	3.4	254

ITEM	AMOUNT	FAT GRAMS	CALORIE PTS	CALORIES
NOONER'S DELI:				
Delite Roast Beef on:				
Marble Bread		8	5.2	390
Wheat Bread		8	5.2	390
Vienna Bread		4	2.7	200
Rye Bread		8	4.9	370
Kaiser Roll		6	3.9	290
Onion Bun		5	3.2	240
Hoagie Roll		5	3.2	240
Delite Turkey on:				
Marble Bread		10	5.3	400
Wheat Bread		10	5.3	400
Vienna Bread		6	2.8	210
Rye Bread		10	5.1	380
Kaiser Roll		8	4.0	300
Onion Bun		7	3.3	250
Hoagie Roll		7	3.3	250
Delight French Dip		6	3.6	270
Fresh Garden Salad		1	0.8	61
Vegetarian Sandwich		10	5.5	413
THE OVEN/LINCOLN-JAIPUR/OMAHA:				
Naan		2	2.6	197
Roti		2	2.7	204
Stuffed Paratha		3	3.2	243
Onion Kulcha		2	2.8	212
Fish Tikka w/Soup & Salad		5	3.7	278
Chicken Tikka Naan w/Soup & Salad		7	5.8	437
Chicken Curry w/Rice, Soup, & Salad (Average)		15	6.7	502
Mixed Vegetable Curry w/Rice		11	5.6	423
Maah Dal w/Rice, Soup, & Salad		12	5.4	406
Bombay Dal w/Rice, Soup, & Salad		9	9.3	697
Raita		0.3	0.9	67

OMAHA A'FARE OF THE HEART
Lincoln & Omaha Restaurants (continued)

ITEM	AMOUNT	FAT GRAMS	CALORIE PTS	CALORIES
The Oven/Lincoln-Jaipur/Omaha (continued):				
Lassi (Average)	0.5		2.2	163
Malai Seekh Kabab w/Rice				
& Salad	8		4.4	330
Chicken Jalfrazie w/Rice & Salad	12		6.3	474
Chicken Vindaloo w/Rice & Salad	15		6.4	481
Chicken Tikka Masala w/ Rice				
& Salad	10		6.2	468
Vegetable Jafrazie w/Rice & Salad	10		4.7	353
Bombay Dal	2.5		1.7	124

PASTA AMORE:
LUNCH

ITEM	AMOUNT	FAT GRAMS	CALORIE PTS	CALORIES
Tomato Salad	0		0.3	24
Leo's Salad	2		0.6	48
Minestrone Soup Cup	1		1.3	100
Pasta w/Tuna Red Sauc and Salad	6		8.9	664
Pasta w/Marinara Sauce and Salad	2		4.8	359

DINNER

ITEM	AMOUNT	FAT GRAMS	CALORIE PTS	CALORIES
Eggplant Parmigiana	2		1.0	77
Chicken Piccata w/Vegetable &				
Pasta w/ Marinara Sauce	7		3.8	282
Chicken Marsala w/ Vegetable				
and Pasta w/Marinara Sauce	7		5.0	378

SPECIALS

ITEM	AMOUNT	FAT GRAMS	CALORIE PTS	CALORIES
Linguine Primavera w/Salad	7		5.6	417
Chicken Primavera w/Salad	10		7.4	557
Spaghetti Puttanesca w/Salad	9		5.5	413
Linguine Gari Baldi w/Salad	12		6.1	454
Linguine Da Vinci w/Salad	16		6.5	488
Mostaccioli Alfio w/Salad	10		8.4	629
Grilled Chicken Dinner w/Vegetable				
Baked Potato, Past w/Marinara,				
& Salad	5		4.6	343

OMAHA A'FARE OF THE HEART
Lincoln & Omaha Restaurants (continued)

ITEM	AMOUNT	FAT GRAMS	CALORIE PTS	CALORIES
THE DELI AT SPIRIT WORLD:				
Fresh Fruit		0.6	0.9	65
Oriental Chicken Salad		6	2.3	172
Italian Chicken Salad		4	1.6	123
Black Bean Soup-				
Cup		3	1.7	126
Bowl		4	2.2	166
Ham & Bean Soup-				
Cup		3	1.7	126
Bowl		4	2.2	165
Minestrone Soup-				
Cup		1	0.5	39
Bowl		2	0.7	52
Vegetable Soup-				
Cup		1	0.5	40
Bowl		2	0.7	52
Chicken Veggie Soup-				
Cup		2	1.0	73
Bowl		3	1.3	95
Beef Barley Soup-				
Cup		2	1.0	76
Bowl		2	1.3	100
Beef Noodle Soup-				
Cup		2	1.4	104
Bowl		3	1.8	137
Sicilian Chicken Breast		8	3.3	251
Grilled Chicken Breast		4	2.8	207
Grilled Chicken Breast				
w/Plum Sauce		4	3.8	285
Chicken Kabobs		8	4.4	329
Biscoti Cookies		5	1.9	139
French Rolls & Loaves: 1 Ounce		0.3	1.1	80

Patient Weight Graph

Patient's Name _____ Date of Program Start _____

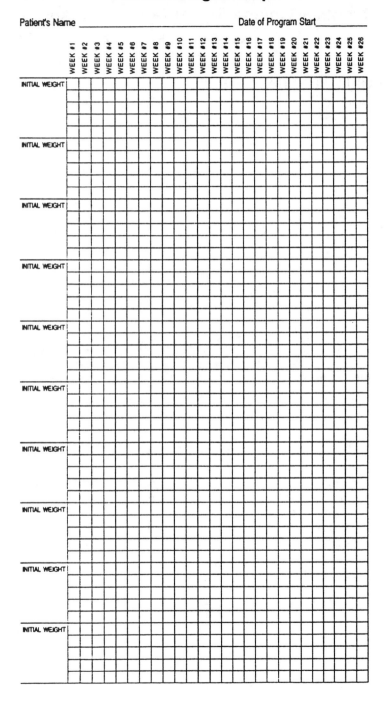

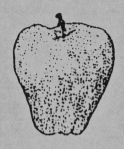

QUICK MENUS FOR FAST AND HEALTHY EATING

Tools to Teach You!

The Menu samples given are beginning places for meals you could begin to experiment with. (with your own personal changes). For years people have asked for menus,and when we started doing some it usually did not last. Yet any use of menus is probably a savings in your bank of fat and calorie intake..,Use these ideas as a beginning of a system that you develop. Menus should be a part of your next grocery list if they are to be helpful. **People with "eating amnesia"-mindless eating ,** can keep on task. with any type of menu/or food plan.

The log sheets are our standbys for people wanting to really learn patterns.You can create a simpler log sheet with 4-5 important focus areas to control, including an avgerage column if this is over a week's time.

Example:	Mon	Tues	Wed	Thurs	AVG
Fat Grams					
Cal Points					
Exercise Min					
Accomplishments					

Experiment with your planner pad or calendar in recording successes and problem areas.No Guilt, just a place to learn.

Karen's Klues: Keeping logs is easy to forget. Total up your numbers before the last meal of the day to save fat and calories overall.. Those who are successful keeping points or fat grams in range usually learn them so well, they can estimate what they've eaten at any time of the day.

QUICK MENUS FOR FAST AND HEALTHY EATING:

Eight breakfasts with 5-10 fat grams:

1 oz canadian bacon	1oz. raisin bran	2 lowfat muffins	1Tpeanut b.
english muffin	toast	Juice	toast
fat free cheese	skim milk	jelly/lt marg	skim milk
juice	lt marg/jelly	hot tea	
banana			
SF hot choc			

2 cinnamon tsts	1sl. banana bread	blueberry bagel	scram. egg
lt marg	f.f. cream cheese	ff cream cheese	toast, lt marg
fresh fruit cup	juice	fresh orange	ff gr turke
skim milk	choc. sk. milk	sk. milk	orange jce

To increase food if these breakfasts do not hold you, double one carbohydrate source, or skim milk first. If still not enough increase one ounce of lean protein(turkey, ham, egg beater, lite cheese)

Eight Lunches with 10-15 fat grams:

Chili Soup*	Deli Turkey Sandwich**	Chicken Taco**	Brocc/Cheese^
Crackers	Baby Carrots	Fresh Apple	Baked Potato
Peach Sl^^	Sugar Free Gelatin w/	FF SF Yogurt	Fresh Grapes
1Sugar Cookie	Fruit	Milk	Toast/lt.marg

Stuffed Tomato#	Roast Beef Sandwich**	Canned Tomato	Hamburger**
w/ tuna/celery/c.ch	Nat. Cnned Fruit Cup	Pasta Gard. Soup	/Bun
W. Wht Crackers	Pretzels	Garlic Tst ##	Fresh Veg's
Strawberries	Vanilla Soft Serve	Fruit Shake ***	Choc. Pudd

*use drained, rinsed lean beef or turkey
**lean to fatfree ingredients used
^fatfree cheese, or light velveeta to give light cheese flavor, increase garlic,etc.
#light mayo/waterpacked tuna/1% or less cottage cheese
##lt on margarine
***2 soft fts/1 ctn ff sf yogurt/milk/ice vanilla(i.e. strawberries, l/2 bananaetc

Men and Active females can double or one and one half servings of entree. Others needing more food simply double carbohydrate sources for more filling effect

Eight Dinners with 15-20 fat grams:

Spaghetti**	Hobo Dinner*	Grilled Halibut	Pork Chop**
Marinara	Rhodes Wheat	Rice w/Mushrooms	Bk Apples/
Pasta	Roll	Broccoli	Onions
Mixed Veg's	Fzn Fruit Mixture	Poached Pears^^	Corn
Brd Sticks		Bran Muffin**	Peach Crisp^
Chicken Noodle	Lasagna**	Beef/Snow Peas**	Gr.Chicken
Soup	Tossed Salad	Rice Stir Fry	Breast/Seas.
French Bread	Green Beans	Parmesan Wht Toast	Pasta
Fruit Bowl	Lite Brownies	Cherry Van. Parfait***	Calif Mix Veg

*4 oz. lean beef cut, potatosliced, l/2onion/carrot pieces in foil with aujus bake one hour,etc...

**lean meat only 3-4 oz portion

^^Fresh pears,mwave w/ orange j. conc and vanilla combo/serve hot or cold

^decrease fat and sugar in recipe by l/3

***lite cherries or lite cherry fllng on ff van. pudding/ van wafer layered combo..Men and active females can increase entrees by one and one half servings, and double one carbohydrate.

Eight Fast Food Menus Avg 10-15 fat grams

Arby's Reg.	Wendy' Gr.	McDonald's Chic.	K.F.C. Rotisserie
Rst. Beef	Chicken	Fajita (2)	Gold Chicken
Sm. Shake	Baked Potato Lite**	Tossed Salad/**	1/4 White w/skin
Salad/Lite	Cup of Chili	Apple Bran Muffin	Mashed Pot/Gravy
Dressing			Corn on the cob
Runza's Gr.	Subway's Turkey	Boston Mkt's	Blimpies Rst. Bf.
Chicken	or Bf	Ham Sandw.	or Turkey 6"
Salad	6 " Whole Wheat	Steamed Veg.	Salad w/fat free
Ch. Noodle Soup	Sandw.		Dressing
	Pretzels		Oat/Raisin Cookie

Eight Snacks averaging 5 fat grams

Rais. Bran Cer.	TurkeySandw*	Pretzels	Tomato Juice
Sk. Milk	Sliced Apple	Fted Yogurt	Baked Seas. Crax
Toast/lt. marg	Bked 'chips	Fresh Peach	Moz. Cheese Stick
Orange Julius**	Lt Fzn Entree	Popcorn	Lge SF Choc Milk
Crackers	Grapes	Free & Clear^	Graham crackers
Frsh Veg/FF Dip	Pasta Salad^^	Peach Jello/fruit	Baked Tostitos
Sm. Juice Spritzer	1/2 Eng. muffin	Pretzels	FF Cheese
	Ice Tea/Lemon		Salsa

**O. J. Conc/Ice/ Vanilla/Sk. Milk,blend
^Walmart Flavored Juice Drinks
^^FF or Lt may/vegetables/pasta w/parmesan, seas.

My Health Count Plan For Today

Day/Date:_____

1.

2.

3.   Delays Used:

Food	Amount	Fat Grams	Cal. Points

Thoughts on the Day	Total:	Total:	Total:

Activity — 5 Minutes Per Block

Type of Activity:

My Health Count Plan For Today

Day/Date:_____

1.

2.

3.   Delays Used:

Food	Amount	Fat Grams	Cal. Points

Thoughts on the Day	Total:	Total:	Total:

Activity — 5 Minutes Per Block

Type of Activity:

Nutrition Matters
Food Score Card

This score card is a quick tool to look at your food intake, a day at a time-for general healthy eating. To understand your own eating patterns, use this food score card 2-3 times weekly. A score of 55 or more could be an initial goal with gradual increases as you replace unnecessary foods and calories with high carbohydrate , healthy choices...

Maximum Score for Each Group		Number of Possible Points	Your Score	DAY:
20	**Milk Group:**			
	I glass/serv	10		
	2 glasses/serv	17		
	3 glasses/serv	20		
20	**Vegetable Group:**			
	1 potato	5		
	1 gr. leafy or yellow	10		
	1 other	5		
20	**Fruit Group:**			
	1 fruit or juice	5		
	2 fts or juices	10		
	1 citrus ft or juice	10		
20	**Bread,Cereal, Pasta Group:**			
	2 servings of any	10		
	4 servings of any	15		
	6 or more servings	20		
15	**Meat Group, Egg, Meat Alternate:**			
	1 serving	l0		
	2 -3 servings	15		
5	**Water:**			
	32 oz. or more	5		

First: ADD THESE FOR A SUB TOTAL   _____

Second: Subtract 5 points for each non or low nutrient food after you have had one for the day(first serving is ok) I.E. 3 large cookies, subtract 10 points for #2 & #3 - _____

Third: Add a score of 5 points for eating something in each food group

+ _____

*Fourth:*Add a score of 5 points if you ate 2 or more servings of the food group that is your least favorite   +_____

TOTAL: _____

At Nutrition Matters, Karen Benson, R.D.C.N. provides individual, groups, and companies nutrition / weight loss counseling as well as these resources. Call us if you have any questions.

Order your copy today!

ε

How To Eat Healthy Wherever You Are
(5th edition of Count For Your Health)   ____copies @ $7.99 ea.   = $_____

Doris Cross Cookbook Vol. 1
(1st edition of fat free &
 ultra lowfat recipes)   ____copies @ $12.95 ea. = $_____

Doris Cross Cookbook Vol. 2
(2nd edition of fat free &
 ultra lowfat recipes)   ____copies @ $12.95 ea. = $_____

Subtotal   ____copies   = $_____

Tax (6% of total)   = $_____

Postage			
How To Eat Healthy Wherever You Are:	1 add $1.47	2-5 add $1.52	
	6-8 add $1.57	9-10 add $1.63	
Doris Cross Cookbooks:	1-2 add $1.52	3-4 add $1.57	= $_____

Total   = $_____

Name_____

Address_____

Phone_____

Make checks payable to: Nutrition Matters
                          PO Box 5253
                          Grand Island, NE 68802
                          Phone (308)381-8361
                          Fax (308)381-8860-0

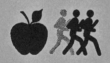

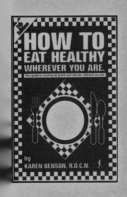

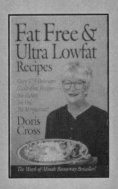

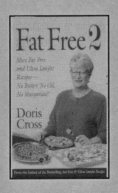